Spiritual Care at the Crossroads

Studies in Spiritual Care

Edited by
Simon Peng-Keller, Eckhard Frick,
Christina Puchalski and John Swinton

Volume 15

Spiritual Care at the Crossroads

Towards a Common Vision for the Future of Christian Healthcare Chaplaincy

Edited by
Simon Peng-Keller, Fabian Winiger and David Neuhold

DE GRUYTER

Published with the support of the Swiss National Science Foundation.

Swiss National
Science Foundation

ISBN 978-3-11-914742-2
e-ISBN (PDF) 978-3-11-220583-9
e-ISBN (EPUB) 978-3-11-220617-1
ISSN 2511-8838
DOI https://doi.org/10.1515/9783112205839

Library of Congress Cataloging-in-Publication Data
A CIP catalog record for this book has been applied for at the Library of Congress.

Bibliographic information published by the Deutsche Nationalbibliothek
The Deutsche Nationalbibliothek lists this publication in the Deutsche Nationalbibliografie; detailed bibliographic data are available on the internet at http://dnb.dnb.de.

Typesetting: Integra Software Services Pvt. Ltd.
Printing and binding: CPI books GmbH, Leck

www.degruyterbrill.com
Questions about General Product Safety Regulation:
productsafety@degruyterbrill.com

MIX
Papier | Fördert gute Waldnutzung
FSC® C083411
FSC www.fsc.org

Preface

This book is the result of a research initiative that responds to the need to clarify the profile of Christian healthcare chaplaincy under the changing conditions of healthcare and society. The increasing complexity, specialization, and digitalization of healthcare, the decline in church resources, the growing pluralization of spiritual and religious practice, and the implementation of interprofessional spiritual care are changing the context of Christian chaplaincy in healthcare and challenge it in many ways.

To clarify these questions and examine possible answers, the editors of this volume invited an international group of experts who for many years have contributed to international debates on spiritual care from a Christian perspective. Attention was paid to bringing together researchers from different countries and different denominational backgrounds and theological approaches. The participants were presented with a series of questions (see Introduction) and asked to write a response in advance of a planned workshop. These contributions were then discussed in depth at the workshop, held over several days in June 2023 in Morschach, Switzerland. Each participant was also invited to present a response to one of the contributions. The aim of this workshop was twofold: on the one hand, we aimed to write a joint White Paper based on our discussions; on the other hand, we hoped to provide the basis for further developing the contributions and ultimately publish them in the present form.

Like the White Paper (Peng-Keller et al. 2025), this volume aims to stimulate critical discussion among all those committed to renewing healthcare chaplaincy in a time of rapid change. This book is an invitation for reflection, discussion, and critical debate to explore a more inclusive form of Christian chaplaincy – one which is sensitive to differences without returning to a narrow confessionalism or an undifferentiated, neutral conception of spirituality and spiritual belonging. It articulates a shared vision for the future of Christian healthcare chaplaincy which contributes to a better healthcare by expanding, deepening, and completing medical practice.

References

Peng-Keller, Simon, Michael Balboni, Tracy Balboni, et al. 2025. "Spiritual Care at the Crossroads: An Ecumenical White Paper on the Future of Christian Healthcare Chaplaincy." *Journal of Religion and Health* 64 (2): 1031–46. https://doi.org/10.1007/s10943-025-02255-0.

https://doi.org/10.1515/9783112205839-202

Contents

Simon Peng-Keller, Fabian Winiger, David Neuhold

Introduction: Healthcare Chaplaincy in a Time of Transition

If there is one point of consensus within current discussions on healthcare chaplaincy, then it is that this is a profession in the midst of a far-reaching transformation process. Healthcare chaplaincy is "surfing through a sea change" (Massey 2014, 144–52). Opinions differ in the analysis and description of this change. Looking more closely, at least two independent processes of change can be identified, which influence each other in complex ways. The first concerns Western societies at large, and is associated with (post-)secularization, religious diversification, and spiritual hybridization. For Christian healthcare chaplaincy, this means partially a decrease in financial and human resources as well as political influence, but also a re-location into a field that is becoming more diverse in religious-spiritual terms. This first process of change is distinct from a second one that has its origin in healthcare itself. It consists, to put it simply, in the expansion of the biopsychosocial health model to include a spiritual dimension. In this context, chaplaincy faces the challenge of clarifying its contribution to healthcare. Part of this process is a reevaluation of the Clinical Pastoral Education (CPE) paradigm, and the development of (a more) outcome-oriented chaplaincy (Massey 2014, 144–52).

From a *longue durée* perspective, the second process of change emerged as early as the first decades of the 20th century. The development of CPE in 1925 by the protestant theologian Anton Boisen and the haematologist Richard Cabot was already a response to modern medicine. These two pioneers had very different ideas about what clinical chaplaincy is and should do. But they shared their protestant background and a common agenda: to include chaplaincy as a unique profession in modern healthcare (Myers-Shirk 2009). In the second half of the 20th century, these two processes of change mentioned entered into a close interplay.[1] The effort to incorporate the spiritual dimension into palliative care and the World Health Organization's "Health for All"-initiative in the 1970s and 1980s was not only directed against an increasingly narrow, reductionistic health care paradigm, but was also informed by an awareness of religious-spiritual diversity (Peng-Keller, Winiger, and Rauch 2022). In these contexts, the appeal to a 'spiritual dimension' of health served to "describe experiences and denote positions and aspirations that are 'more than' or 'move beyond' either secularity or religion" (Bender and Taves 2012, 6). In this usage, the term 'spiritual' both presupposes

1 Cf. the documents quoted in Cadge (2019).

https://doi.org/10.1515/9783112205839-001

and transcends the religious/secular duality typical for modernity in general, and modern medicine in particular (Berger 2015, 410).

For *Christian* healthcare chaplaincy, these processes of change result in several challenging questions that are addressed in this volume. As a basis for our discussion, we identified four areas where these changes have profoundly challenged its practitioners:

1. The dual role of "representative of a (specific) faith community" and "specialized health professional"[2] in secular health systems: How can the tension between this dual role and belonging of Christian chaplains be made fruitful under the conditions of today's health care system(s) and pluralistic societies? What is the role of healthcare chaplaincy in the broader context of the Christian involvement in healthcare?
2. Medical goals and the "Christian call to health and healing": To which medical goals can Christian healthcare chaplaincy contribute? What does "spiritual healing" mean in the context of healthcare chaplaincy? What does the ecumenical reflection on the enduring biblical "call to health and healing" mean for the task of healthcare chaplains?
3. Personal spiritual practice(s) and professionalism: What is the impact of the personal spiritual rootedness of chaplains for professional spiritual care, and how can it be integrated into education, training, and evaluation? What is the role of spirituality and theology in future chaplaincy formation?
4. A paradigm shift within CPE: Does the emphasis on "outcomes" in current chaplaincy research (and other factors, e.g. digitalization, pluralization, secularization) lead to a (paradigm) shift within chaplaincy formation and training, especially in CPE (cf. Hall, Handzo, and Massey 2026)? To what extent is a "presence orientation" compatible with a stronger reflection on professional objectives in the field of spiritual care?

As the contributions in this volume demonstrate, an answer to these questions must take into account different national contexts and historical circumstances. The differences concern both the training and commissioning of healthcare chaplains and the legal framework and funding of their employment. While in the Netherlands, the United Kingdom, and in Northern America, healthcare chaplains are financed by the state or by the health care system, in Germany and Switzer-

2 The difference between spiritual care generalists and spiritual care specialists has become widely accepted in the course of the first decade of the new millennium, cf. Handzo and Koenig (2004).

land they are largely – although probably not for too much longer – church funded.

In addition, there are historical and social factors. Even where the funding and the structural framework are similar, healthcare chaplains may find themselves in remarkably different situations. A comparison between chaplaincy in the NHS England and the NHS Scotland is instructive.[3] In both countries, the current policy on healthcare chaplaincy was set by secular governments around the millennium (Swift 2014), and in both cases the principle of equality was central for the attempt to organize the profession (NHS England 2020; EHRC 2023). But the paths chosen went in opposite directions. While in England the New Labour government sought to reflect the religious diversity of society in chaplaincy teams, the Scottish government laid the foundations for a spiritual care that is strictly separated from religious backgrounds and practices. Now, more than twenty years later, it has become apparent: Both paths produce considerable challenges that will be discussed throughout this volume. Let us consider the critical analysis of Scottish chaplain Duncan MacLaren to which several of the contributions in this book will refer (MacLaren 2021).[4]

The challenges of the denominational approach opted by the NHS England, he argues, are threefold: First, it pursues an unrealistic goal. MacLaren states succinctly that "in a highly diverse context with a small chaplaincy team, the cake can only be cut in so many ways" (MacLaren 2021, 29). Even a large chaplaincy team can at best only represent the main faith communities, never all of them, and never all their variants. Since the English model assumes clear faith identities and fixed denominational affiliations, it fails to represent not only smaller communities, but also the growing number of those who are unaffiliated or whose religious and spiritual attitudes and affiliations are fluid. Inevitably, the New Labour approach towards greater equality becomes discriminatory against minority groups outside and within the dominant religious communities.

Second, the English multi-denominational approach remains wedded to the notion that the primary task of chaplaincy is explicitly religious and best performed by commissioned representatives of religious communities. Without intending, it "perpetuates the perception among clinical staff that chaplaincy teams are mostly there to provide religious care for the faithful, rather than spiritual care for all – a perception that can lead to inequitable access to spiritual care for those of no specific faith or belief" (MacLaren 2021, 29).

3 See the contributions of Chris Swift and John Swinton in this volume.
4 See Anne Vandenhoeck's and John Swinton's chapter in this volume.

Finally, this approach does not foster the integration of chaplains in interprofessional teams. Focusing on religious and ideological diversity in the structuring of healthcare chaplaincy leads to a different care logic and prioritization than if the focus is determined by clinical-therapeutic criteria and the goal is to implement spiritual care as interprofessionally as possible.

The challenges of the generic approach chosen by NHS Scotland are no less intricate: First, the separation between 'spiritual care' and 'religious care' is conceptually artificial and empirically questionable. It corresponds neither to the history of concepts nor to current research, which demonstrates a strong terminological overlap.

Second, this separation is difficult to sustain in everyday clinical practice and is unlikely to meet the needs of patients in many cases. It is not best practice for a spiritual caregiver to call on an external colleague to perform a ritual that s/he could carry out him-/herself.

Third, the generic approach strains the integrity and authenticity of chaplains as spiritual caregiver and fosters "a withdrawal from theological reflection upon the work of the chaplain" (MacLaren 2021, 34).

The diverging developments in the United Kingdom exemplify similar trends in other countries. To name but two examples: The development in Canada, where it is now possible to become a state-recognized *Certified Practitioner of Spiritual Care* (O'Connor and Meakes 2021), is similar to that in Scotland, while the English policy is reminiscent of the Dutch regulation of healthcare chaplaincy via different sections.[5] Looking at developments in Western Europe, North America, Australia and New Zealand, a common pattern emerges regardless of the various differences: The 'old order' of healthcare chaplaincy determined by strong Christian institutions is replaced increasingly by new ones which compel Christian healthcare chaplaincy to radically reorient itself. How can it be positioned in such a way that the aforementioned problems are avoided?

Congruent with many of the contributions to this volume, MacLaren delineates a third way, beyond the multi-denominational and the generic approach. It is based on the assumption that chaplains, by virtue of their training and personal practice, are shaped by a particular spiritual tradition. Their particular belonging and formation are one of many pathways to a common professional identity that is inclusive for other traditions. According to MacLaren, spiritual traditions fulfil a formative function for healthcare chaplaincy that can be compared to that of the schools of psychotherapy. Psychotherapists, like chaplains, practice in a particular modality: "Competence in working within one's core mo-

5 See the contribution of Wim Smeets to this book.

dality is a prerequisite for practice [...] having no 'spiritual modality' is not an option [...] a chaplain is precisely someone who has been formed within a particular wisdom tradition (Jewish, Buddhist, Sikh, Humanist, and so forth), and has developed the critical skills to be able to draw upon the resources of that tradition, and to critique its weaknesses. [...] it is this rootedness in the spirituality of one or more concrete, historical, wisdom traditions that makes chaplains distinctive and constitutes their 'unique selling point'" (MacLaren 2021, 36).

One could deepen MacLaren's analogy with the aid of psychotherapy research that proves the personal relationship as the decisive therapeutic factor. The methods, which are important for the professional identity, are effective *insofar* they enable safe and therapeutic relationships between therapists and clients. The same may be said of the formative traditions of healthcare chaplaincy: They are helpful *insofar* they enable spiritual care givers to build supportive relationships with people in distress (patients, relatives, professionals). In this way, it is also possible to answer the question that repeatedly arose in the discussions among the authors of this book when it came to the question of the double affiliation of chaplains.

Expressed with a comparison from football: When chaplains are mandated by both their faith communities and health care institutions, what is the leg to stand on and what is the free leg to play? To embody[6] a spiritual tradition and bring it into a professional activity, one must stand in it and live from it, and not just formally belong to it. Their spiritual 'footing' and embodied practices give healthcare chaplains the freedom to engage flexibly and professionally in changing clinical environments and interpersonal constellations.

The contributions collected in this volume outline different, partly converging, but sometimes also diverging ways of responding to the situation outlined on the preceding pages. While all authors agree that the concept of a generic chaplaincy is problematic, there are considerable differences in how the particular anchoring in a specific tradition should align with the task of accompanying people with very diverse convictions and affiliations. The following approaches range from "cooperative pluralism" (Baker 2021) to the art of reflective code-switching (Cadge and Sigalow 2013) and the self-transformative adventure of theological and spiritual hospitality (Youngblood 2019; Jyothi and Susan 2024).

The first chapter, contributed by one of the editors, presents an argument in four steps, and clarifies it with a case report. First, it is argued, the renewal of Christian healthcare chaplaincy requires the rediscovery of the "call to healing"

6 Cf. Daniel Nuzum's differentiation (this volume): "As a specialised spiritual carer, [...] the Christian healthcare chaplain embodies their tradition and faith, rather than being a performer of it."

found in the synoptic Gospels, as well as a clarification of the therapeutic dimension of spiritual care. Second, this call is primarily met in sharing responsibility for a holistic and just healthcare by using all available methods to (trans-)form secular healthcare from within. Third, this goal can only be reached through interprofessional collaboration, and chaplains participate in this task as specialists in spiritual care who are subject to an "ethic of accountability". Fourth, healthcare chaplaincy contributes to secular healthcare precisely through its spiritual character, which has several aspects and should not be reduced to just one.

In the second chapter, Anne Vandenhoeck takes issue with the fact that more and more people in Western societies do not identify with organized religions or belief systems. Should chaplains follow suit? And should those with a spiritual tradition hide it to become "chameleons", adapting to the spirituality of those in front of them? There are a fluidity and universality in spiritual care. A comparison made by MacLaren (2021) states there are common characteristics in therapy. However, therapists have schools, and chaplains should have a spiritual identity tied to a spiritual tradition. There is no such thing as neutrality as chaplains need their spiritual self to do spiritual care. In this contribution, Anne Vandenhoeck advocates for spiritual caregivers' rootedness in spiritual traditions in the midst of ongoing processes of secularization, pluralization, and detraditionalization. How can chaplains be authentic in spiritual care for patients against the background of a decreased value of a spiritual identity based on a spiritual tradition? An exploration of integrity and authenticity is needed to understand the communication about identity in spiritual caregiving. There is great variety in the prominence of the spiritual identity of the chaplain in relation to the patient. However, she argues, it is of importance to the quality of spiritual care. Creating space for the patient's spirituality requires expert handling of one's own spiritual identity without denying it.

In the next chapter, Michael and Tracy Balboni argue that Christian healthcare chaplaincy is founded on Christ himself – his life, teachings, and healings as well as his death and resurrection. His repeated words spoken in the context of his healings «Your faith has made you well» provide a framework for Christian spiritual care and the goals of Christian healing. These words embody the source of healing, the process by which healing takes place, and the goal to which Christian healing is directed. Employing theological reflection and a patient case, this chapter aims to illuminate this Christ-entered framework and illustrate how it informs Christian spiritual care in the medical setting. Accordingly, Christian healthcare chaplaincy is sourced in faith in the triune God, centred on personal and communal practices of restoring wholeness and directed to ultimate wholeness found in Christ.

The following contribution by Annette Haußmann reflects on the current transformation processes within hospital chaplaincy in Germany, drawing insights from case vignettes of pastoral care practice. It highlights tensions between hospital chaplaincy as specialized pastoral care and parish related pastoral care, emphasizing the need to conceptualize the health-promoting dimension of pastoral care more broadly as part of congregational work and a community-oriented church. Particular potentials lie in outpatient care, especially given the reduced hospital stays and the increasing need for measures of health prevention. An interprofessionally connected hospital chaplaincy can provide valuable input in this context. This chapter argues that there is a need to foster empirical research on hospital chaplaincy, to enhance knowledge about its effectiveness and role in healthcare. In an environment primarily driven by empirical evidence and efficacy in hospital economics, hospital chaplaincy must position itself transparently and confidently, with high-quality empirical research playing a crucial role. Emphasizing the importance of a detailed focus on lived spirituality is particularly important, including the perspective of healthcare chaplains in shaping their personal and professional identity. Looking ahead, this chapter addresses the future challenges and opportunities, discussing the concept of "outreaching chaplaincy" and the prospective financing of healthcare chaplaincy.

The past thirty years, argues Chris Swift subsequently, have witnessed social and religious transformation at an unprecedented pace. In health care, this has led to a rapid diversification in the professional providers of spiritual care, ranging from an ever-increasing number of faiths to the emergence of provision by practitioners who are not religious. All of this reflects a decline in religious identification in the population at large, evidenced by national censuses. Drawing on a case study involving a Humanist chaplain and faith-identified colleagues, the challenges and opportunities of work in this new reality are discussed. The experience of using a more sensitive tool to capture complex patient religion/belief identity is described and explored. In considering this approach, it is recognised that a move away from simple (census-like) categories may produce information which has a) greater accuracy but also, b) contradictory and fragmentary data. Based on these discussions, proposals are made relating to training; employers; and the provision of spiritual care to individuals and groups that are neurodiverse. Finally, theological consideration is given to Christian chaplaincy practice in the rapidly changing landscape of spirituality. In contexts of intensifying diversity and complexity, skilled and knowledgeable Christian chaplains have much to offer in helping people negotiate their beliefs within the experience of illness.

In the next chapter, Trace Haythorn argues that Christian healthcare chaplaincy has the potential to be a central form of religious leadership in the twenty-first century; however, multiple tensions exist within and without the profession that hinder its impact and its self-understanding. Drawing on his decade-long experience as the director of the American Association for Clinical Pastoral Education (ACPE), he explores several of these tensions, striving to identify and, when possible, disentangle the complexities of chaplaincy practice, formation, and profession.

The next chapter, contributed by Daniel Nuzum, outlines the development of healthcare chaplaincy in Ireland from a primarily religious expression and provision towards a broader pluralistic approach. This development is traced alongside the changing demographics of Irish society and the growing recognition of the development of healthcare chaplaincy as a profession. The evolving dual relationship of the Christian healthcare chaplain to their faith community and to the healthcare institution is illustrated as a creative liminal space. Drawing on a case study of a baby diagnosed with a congenital fetal anomaly, the chapter illustrates how Christian healthcare chaplaincy' has much to contribute to professional spiritual care in a pluralist context. The contribution of Clinical Pastoral Education (CPE) to the education and formation of healthcare chaplains/spiritual carers is outlined. CPE in Ireland continues to develop as a competency-based approach with international reciprocity. The developments in CPE as an integrative process are congruent with developments in wider healthcare education and the scholarship of teaching and learning. These developments in practice, approach, and education recognize the importance of the spiritual identity of the healthcare chaplain and their place as the spiritual care expert on the interdisciplinary healthcare team.

Traugott Roser, in the following chapter, argues that pastoral care – in its essence – is a meaningful encounter between two or more people sharing experience, burdens and needs, emotions, and resources of faith, hope, and love in a situation of vulnerability. What makes these encounters Christian is the possibility that Christ's presence can be recognised in hindsight, by reflecting on them through Scripture. This chapter reflects on the author's personal pathways as healthcare chaplain and as receiver of spiritual care, and theoretically framed models for future specialized spiritual care as part of a multiprofessional team. It covers aspects of training in the tradition of CPE, the importance of academic theological education, interdisciplinary research, and the moral dimension of spiritual care. One part of being a chaplain is artful use of skills and technique; the other part is personal experience based in both individual spiritual life and lived Christian faith. Christian healthcare chaplains belong to two living bodies, linking the body of Christ and the functional organism that is the healthcare system.

What does spiritual healing mean? In the next chapter, John Swinton grapples with the concepts of spirituality and spiritual healing as multifaceted and complex concepts. The chapter suggests that the lack of a universal definition is not a sign of meaninglessness, but rather an indication of the complexity and socially constructed nature of spiritual experiences. Spirituality is presented as a quest to address four existential questions: Who am I? Where do I come from? Where am I going? And why? These questions gain prominence in the face of illness and suffering and have traditionally been answered within the frameworks of world religions. In the post-religious, highly individualised Western society, spirituality has evolved into a more personal and less communally shared pursuit. Individuals seek answers to life's bigger questions through personal hopes, desires, and cultural expectations, rather than through religious narratives. The chapter considers spirituality as a generic term, not tied to any specific religion or belief system, but rather a broad concept that can encompass various forms of expression and individual searches for meaning. The concept of "relational consciousness" as defined by David Hay and Rebecca Nye, argues Swinton, proposes an innate human predisposition toward spiritual experience, observable in the unadulterated spirituality of children. Their qualitative research supports the hypothesis that humans are hard-wired for spirituality, a sense of awe, and wonder, suggesting that spirituality may be a universal, generic human need rather than merely a cultural artifact. This chapter contrasts the impact of cultural milieu on the nature of spirituality, comparing collectivist cultures with the individualized Western perspective. In the West, spiritual needs and experiences are often centred around the self, focusing on personal meaning and self-actualisation.

In the final chapter, Wim Smeets shows how spiritual care in the Netherlands has undergone enormous development over the last half century, closely linked to the changed world-view landscape in society. Not only do people draw from multiple sources for their spirituality, spiritual caregivers do so themselves. A new group of spiritual caregivers has emerged who cannot or do not want to receive a mission from a church or other world-view organizations, but who receive a mandate from an independent council for non-institutionally bound spiritual caregivers. A case study illustrates how spiritual competency and spiritual care competency apply to these new spiritual caregivers and how they relate to their church colleagues. This development towards more autonomy is not at odds, but actually in line with, the development of Christian spirituality. This also has consequences for CPE as the most important further training for spiritual caregivers worldwide.

Taken together, these contributions — written by many of the leading contemporary voices on Christian spiritual care — share way markers in personal and professional journeys, moments for pause and critical self-reflection, as well as new horizons of healing and inspiration amidst the ongoing transforming of healthcare chaplaincy as it faces rapid and increasingly uncertain societal transformations. Drawing on these contributions and the discussions at the workshop in Morschach, a White Paper (Peng-Keller et al. 2025) complements these contributions by gathering and synthesizing the central theological, practical and political challenges raised by the contributors, and offering a clear and hopeful vision for a future healthcare in which chaplains to play a central and indispensable part in holistic, person-centred healthcare.

References

Baker, Alan T. 2021. Foundations of Chaplaincy: A Practical Guide. Michigan: Wm. B. Eerdmans Publishing.

Bender, Courtney, and Ann Taves. 2012. "Introduction: Things of Value." In What Matters?: Ethnographies of Value in a Not So Secular Age, edited by Courtney Bender and Ann Taves, 1–33. New York, NY: Columbia University Press.

Berger, Peter L. 2015. "The Hospital: On the Interface Between Secularity and Religion." Society 52 (5): 410–12. https://doi.org/10.1007/s12115-015-9941-z.

Cadge, Wendy. 2019. "Healthcare Chaplaincy as a Companion Profession: Historical Developments." Journal of Health Care Chaplaincy 25 (2): 45–60. https://doi.org/10.1080/08854726.2018.1463617.

Cadge, Wendy, and Emily Sigalow. 2013. "Negotiating Religious Differences: The Strategies of Interfaith Chaplains in Healthcare." Journal for the Scientific Study of Religion 52 (1): 146–58. https://doi.org/10.1111/jssr.12008.

EHRC. 2023. "Public Sector Equality Duty: Guidance for Public Authorities." Gov.Uk. December 18, 2023. https://www.gov.uk/government/publications/public-sector-equality-duty-guidance-for-public-authorities/public-sector-equality-duty-guidance-for-public-authorities.

Hall, Eric J, George H Handzo, and Kevin Massey. 2026. "Time to Move Forward. A New Model of Spiritual Care to Enhance the Delivery of Outcomes and Value in Health Care Settings." HealthCare Chaplaincy Network.

Handzo, George, and Harold G Koenig. 2004. "Spiritual Care: Whose Job Is It Anyway?" Southern Medical Journal 97 (12): 1242–45. https://doi.org/10/dxbxxz.

Jyothi, Andrew, and Isaac Susan. 2024. "How Shall I Sing the Lord's Song in a Strange Land? Christian Biblical Perspectives on Theological Integrity in Inter- and Multifaith Chaplaincy." In Chaplaincy: Contemporary and Global Perspectives, edited by Grace Thomas and Kim Wasey, 91–104. London: SCM Press.

MacLaren, Duncan. 2021. "All Things to All People? The Integrity of Spiritual Care in a Plural Health Service." Health & Social Care Chaplaincy 9 (1): 27–41.

Massey, Kevin. 2014. "Surfing through a Sea Change: The Coming Transformation of Chaplaincy Training." Reflective Practice: Formation and Supervision in Ministry 1 (0). https://journals.sfu.ca/rpfs/index.php/rpfs/article/view/353.

Myers-Shirk, Susan E. 2009. Helping the Good Shepherd: Pastoral Counselors in a Psychotherapeutic Culture, 1925–1975. Baltimore, MD: Johns Hopkins University Press.

NHS England. 2020. "NHS England and NHS Improvement: Equality and Health Inequalities Impact Assessment (EHIA) Template." NHS England. https://www.england.nhs.uk/wp-content/uploads/2023/08/chaplaincy-guidance-ehia.pdf.

O'Connor, Thomas St. James, and Elizabeth Meakes. 2021. "Three Emerging Spiritual Practices in the Canadian Association for Spiritual Care (CASC): From Pastoral Care and Counselling to Multi-Faith, Evidence-Based Spiritual Care and Psycho-Spiritual Therapy." Journal of Pastoral Care & Counseling 75 (4): 278–83. https://doi.org/10.1177/15423050211036662.

Peng-Keller, Simon, Michael Balboni, Tracy Balboni, Annette Haußmann, Trace Haythorn, Pascal Mösli, David Neuhold, et al. 2025. "Spiritual Care at the Crossroads: An Ecumenical White Paper on the Future of Christian Healthcare Chaplaincy." Journal of Religion and Health, February. https://doi.org/10.1007/s10943-025-02255-0.

Peng-Keller, Simon, Fabian Winiger, and Raphael Rauch. 2022. The Spirit of Global Health: The World Health Organization and the "Spiritual Dimension" of Health, 1946–2021. Oxford, New York: Oxford University Press.

Swift, Christopher. 2014. Hospital Chaplaincy in the Twenty-First Century: The Crisis of Spiritual Care on the NHS. 2nd ed. Explorations in Practical, Pastoral and Empirical Theology. Farnham, Surrey, England: Ashgate.

Youngblood, Peter Ward. 2019. "Interfaith Chaplaincy as Interpretive Hospitality." Religions 10 (3): 226. https://doi.org/10.3390/rel10030226.

Simon Peng-Keller

Answering the Christian Call to Healing. Healthcare Chaplaincy as Specialised Spiritual Care

Abstract: This chapter presents an argument in four steps and clarifies it with a case report. First, it is argued, the renewal of Christian healthcare chaplaincy requires the rediscovery of the "call to healing" found in the synoptic Gospels, as well as a clarification of the therapeutic dimension of spiritual care. Second, this call is primarily met in sharing responsibility for a holistic and just healthcare by using all available methods to (trans-)form secular healthcare from within. Third, this goal can only be reached through interprofessional collaboration, and chaplains participate at this task as specialists in spiritual care who are subject to an "ethic of accountability". Fourth, healthcare chaplaincy contributes to secular healthcare precisely through its spiritual character, which has several aspects and should not be reduced to just one.

My own way into healthcare chaplaincy came unexpected and almost coincidentally. In 1992, I refused compulsory military service and was brought before the court as a conscientious objector. It was the time just before civilian service was introduced in Switzerland as an alternative to compulsory military service. The judges in military uniform sentenced me to seven-month labour in a public institution, a duty that became a state-sponsored chaplaincy internship. After this initiation into healthcare chaplaincy, which included a CPE course, I was involved in chaplaincy in different contexts – in a parish, in assisted living facilities and in contemplative retreats – but it took more than 20 years before I returned to healthcare. In 2016, when I stated to work as a chaplain in a palliative care unit, I realised that the conditions of healthcare chaplaincy in Switzerland had changed to a far greater extent than I had expected.

To give just two examples: As a chaplain in the early 1990s, I had only occasionally participated in nursing rapports in. When I returned to this vocation in 2016, however, I became officially part of the interprofessional team on the palliative care center where I worked. Likewise, as a chaplaincy trainee, I already had the opportunity to inspect the patient files, which at that time consisted of hanging registers. However, I hardly used this opportunity, as the verbal information I received from nursing staff was sufficient for my work. Over two decades later,

https://doi.org/10.1515/9783112205839-002

the old-fashioned registers had disappeared and been replaced by digital patient files. The question of how chaplains should participate in clinical documentation started to be intensively discussed and became the subject of one of the first research projects I was able to conduct at the newly created professorship for Spiritual Care at the University of Zurich (cf. Peng-Keller and Neuhold 2020). This professorship was itself a response to the upheaval in the field of healthcare chaplaincy and the emergence of interprofessional spiritual care, which was recognised by the Swiss Federal Office of Public Health in 2010 as a pillar of palliative care.

All this led to controversies. In German-speaking chaplaincy, the anglicism "spiritual care" was initially met with great suspicion. Many saw it as a keyword for a secularized, dechristianized and medicalized form of healthcare chaplaincy, while others saw it as a welcome opportunity for professionalisation. For me, having been imprinted in the Christian contemplative tradition and Catholic theology of spirituality, this polarised debate offered the challenge to explore ways in which Christian healthcare chaplaincy can use structural changes as an opportunity to renew and raise its profile. Four convictions crystallized for me, which will be further unfolded on the following pages:[1] First, the renewal of Christian healthcare chaplaincy requires a rediscovery of the "call to healing" found in the synoptic Gospels as well as a clarification of the therapeutic dimension of spiritual care. Second, this call is primarily met in sharing responsibility for a holistic and just healthcare by using all available methods to (trans-)form secular healthcare from within. Third, this goal can only be reached through interprofessional collaboration, and chaplains participate in this task as specialists in spiritual care who are subject to an "ethic of accountability". Fourth, healthcare chaplaincy contributes to secular healthcare precisely by its spiritual character, which has several aspects and should not be reduced to just one. A case report will help clarify my argument and relate it to my experience. But let us turn first to the Christian call to healing: Why hark back to this biblical topic?

1 The Christian Call to Healing: A Framework for An Ongoing Commitment

"Our calling to health and healing is as strong as ever" (WCC 2017, para. 3) With this bold affirmation, the *World Council of Churches* in 2017 presented a new

1 For a more detailed account, see Peng-Keller (2024).

Global Ecumenical Health Strategy. This call has a long history behind it, and a strong biblical foundation. According to the synoptic gospels, Jesus called on his disciples not only to preach, but also to heal: "Then Jesus called the twelve together and gave them power and authority over all demons and to cure diseases, and he sent them out to proclaim the kingdom of God and to heal." (Luke 9:1–2).[2] Whatever the meaning of this call, it is rooted in the ministry of Jesus: "Jesus was a healer and exorcist with a special profile that is still recognisable today" (Theißen 2008, 50). The disciples are called to continue a therapeutic task: mediating God's healing presence. And they are called to do it not alone but in cooperation, as they are sent in pairs (Mark 6:7).

What characterizes the healing envisioned in the biblical narratives? To hint at just a few aspects: The healings are embedded in a relationship that unfolds in an unpredictable way. They follow a charismatic impulse, rather than a sapiential logic, as found, for example, in Ben Sira's praise for the good and wise physician (Sirach 38:1–14).[3] With all the diversity of the narrated healings, certain common characteristics nevertheless emerge. Often, though not always, they happen through touch. As much as Jesus may resemble an ancient healer in this respect, he differs in working almost entirely without the usual aids. Neither pharmacological substances nor fixed rituals are employed. In most of the stories, there is not even a healing prayer. Instead, it is the faith and the trust of the sufferers that is of central importance. If anything about Jesus' therapeutic ministry is historically unique, it may be the formula: "Your faith has made you well!" (Luke 17:19) What may appear to be a modest gesture of a humble healer has a peculiar reversal effect: When the healed "attribute the healing power to the healer", Jesus instead "reattributes it – against their expectations – to their faith" (Theißen 2008, 54).

In the course of the long history of Christian interpretation, there have been voices that have regarded the healing mission as an initial phenomenon that has long since been accomplished. The prevailing view, however, is that it is a basic Christian duty that must be answered anew at every time. The question then is not *whether* at all, but *how* exactly. Whatever this means in a complex and highly specialized healthcare system, chaplaincy has a key role to play.

My thesis is: Understanding healthcare chaplaincy as a specific answer to the Christian call to healing grounds and embeds it in two ways. *On the one hand*, this underlines the (in the broad sense) 'therapeutic' dimension of chaplaincy work. It

2 Later Jesus gives the mission to an extended group of Jesus' followers as well and sends them out (Luke 10,9).
3 On this contrast: Jobin (2020).

contributes in its own way to coping with illness and death. Reducing suffering and supporting recovering and healing is not and never has been an exclusively medical task. It is, in any case, not a task that medicine can perform alone. Physicians are and remain dependent on other professions – including that of chaplaincy. If chaplains see themselves in the horizon of the Christian call to healing, they can articulate their contribution to healthcare and healing without submitting to external goals.

On the other hand, chaplaincy is thus put in a broader perspective. It contributes, together with other professionals and volunteers, to an encompassing task: the commitment to just and humane healthcare. No matter how hidden, fleeting and individual the work of chaplains may be – it is thus still part of a community effort. What distinguishes chaplaincy as specialised spiritual care from other ways of answering the Christian call to healing is its particular professional profile. As a specialised profession in healthcare, it operates in clinical contexts which are characterised by a high degree of professionalism and a strong orientation towards scientific evidence. This brings us to the next point.

2 Medical goals and the Christian difference

Healthcare chaplains require a triple mandate: by faith communities, health institutions, and, most importantly, by patients or their relatives. Vested with a triple mandate, they are brokers who mediate between (at least) three highly complex and often tense worlds. Against the background of a spiritual tradition in which they themselves are rooted and which they embody, they engage with the spiritual belief needs of patients and relatives, and they do so within the context of a health institution and in cooperation with health professionals. Their work is driven by a threefold mandate: their own spiritual vocation, the assignment by the health institution and the mandate they receive from patients and relatives.

Under the current conditions, two challenges arise: On the one hand, clarifying the mandate with patients and relatives is an ongoing process that requires communicative fine-tuning. On the other hand, the relationship between the spiritual and the medical perspectives and approaches must be clarified – on a fundamental level as well as in concrete situations where tensions emerge. In the following case report, both challenges can be found. Two longer and two shorter encounters are summarized based on my own clinical documentation.

Mr W. has been referred to the Palliative Care Unit for complex discharge planning and has asked for the chaplain. According to the medical prognosis, he has only a limited life ahead of him; the care team is looking for a free place in a hos-

pice close to his home. I meet him together with his elderly mother, sister and brother-in-law. They all have many questions, especially the mother who expresses fear of loss. Religious belonging is important to all of them. Mr. W. talks about a professional project that he still wants to complete. He feels torn about how to deal with the bad prognosis: Fight or accept? He also says that prayer and receiving communion mean a lot to him. His faith gives him strength and comfort. The hospital stay has slowed him down in a positive way: he used to be impatient, now he has time to think.

At the next meeting, I bring him the Holy Communion and pray the Veni Sancte Spiritus with him. Afterwards, we talk about his current state of health. He is shocked at how emaciated he has become. He does not quite know how to proceed with the question of nutrition. He had refused a feeding tube and forced himself unsuccessfully to ingest the food given to him. If he stops eating, he will probably die quickly, and he does not know if it makes sense to prolong his life. He speaks slowly and with long pauses. He asks me if there are studies that show that people realize when it no longer makes sense to continue to fight in a "situation like that" because of an intuition. Later he gives himself an answer. He feels that he still has a task, namely, to finish the project already mentioned, into which he has put a lot of heart and finances. He had always been religious, but twelve years ago, he experienced a kind of second conversion. He came across videos of healing miracles on the internet and gradually became convinced that such healings were Jesus' current "PR strategy". He became increasingly aware that God really existed and was effectively present in his life. His life project was then given to him three years later in the aftermath of a prayer ritual.

At this moment, a dynamic woman comes in the door. Mr. W. has previously announced her as an important person of reference and now asks her to tell me her story, which she does. Since she herself almost died of an illness a few years ago, she had been given the gift of receiving messages from Jesus. She had been commissioned by him to pray for the healing of sick people and to conduct healing services. She also prayed intensively for Mr. W. and was hopeful that he would get well. In any case, she had not received any message to the contrary. She also explains what she experienced when she laid her hands on him recently. It was imperative that the stomach be reactivated. She turns to Mr W. and urges him to eat regularly again. He refuses; he could no longer ingest the food. The woman, however, does not let up. He must force himself, then it will come again, she reminds him. Mr W. seems disgruntled. She is sometimes quite resolute, she explains her behaviour to me. I interject that the problem is the tumour and that in the end it doesn't matter for a divinely effected healing whether he eats or not. "God wants us to participate in the healing," she replies. And it is also about a positive inner attitude. You must not give up on yourself, but fight. "You have to fight too, A.!" And so it goes on for a while until I finally say goodbye to both of them and promise to come back the next day.

It was not clear to me after the conversation how to deal with the tension I had got into. It was clearly noticeable that Mr W. had a very close relationship with his friend (and maybe partner) and that her support was of central importance to him. At the same time, it was impossible not to notice that her urging burdened Mr W. and that she did not give much space to the questions he was carrying inside. Had it been right to cautiously inquire about her idea of healing and thus move to the theological level? I wanted to offer Mr W. an alternative Christian perspective. But did I succeed? Had I not rather disqualified myself in his eyes by these enquiries, by joining the group of those who met with scepticism the hope for healing that he himself cherished and that his counsellor embodied? Despite these misgivings, I finally decided to ask Mr. W. at the next visit how he had fared with the intervention of his friend. I did not want to miss the opportunity to give more space to the questions he had expressed to me.

I meet Mr W. turned inwards. When I ask him about yesterday's conversation, he admits that his spiritual advisor is "unrealistic" about his diet. The most important thing, however, was his healing. There are very few people like him who are convinced that they can talk directly to Jesus. Unlike the first two visits, the conversation with Mr. W. does not really get going in this encounter. Have I distanced myself from him through my theological discussion with his companion? Or is his reclusiveness simply due to the progression of the disease and an increasing fatigue? I am told by the interprofessional team that his strength was waning, and that Mr. W. seemed increasingly absent.

At the last visit, Mr. W. is very tired and seems sad. For a few brief moments he looks at me quite awake. There is a religious picture on his chest. He had just gone through a long and comforting prayer ritual. I inform him that I will be away for ten days from tomorrow and say goodbye to him. He thanks me for my support. The following Monday, Mr. W. is transferred to a hospice, where he dies three days later.

In this case report, the chaplain joins a family in anticipatory grief. Called up by the patient and welcomed by his relatives, he had no difficulty settling into his role and uniting his three mandates: What the patient and his relatives expected from him was congruent with his spiritual background and the role that he fulfilled within the palliative care team. That the different reference systems, which chaplains are charged with reconciling, by no means interfered without tension became apparent in the second encounter. With the appearance of Mr. W.'s friend, herself a kind of spiritual advisor and possibly also his partner, the constellation changed significantly.

The spiritually based imperative that Mr. W. must fight and eat, which obviously caused him distress, also challenges the chaplain. How should he respond to it? Should he be content with the perception of this tension and return to it at a favourable opportunity? In retrospect, this seems the better path than the one I chose spontaneously. Only in retrospect did I realize how complicated Mr. W's relationship probably was and had ventured into something concerning it. Whether her refusal to accept Mr. W.'s renunciation of food was also based on her own defence against grief, I will never know. It is clear, however, that I could only partially meet the demand to respond to Mr. W.'s ambivalence, his wavering between contradictory inner and outer voices, in the best possible way. I wish I could have given him more space to clarify and validate these voices for himself.

Mr. W.'s physical and emotional suffering was complicated by a spiritual conundrum: Should he still hope for healing, or rather stop struggling and surrender his life to God? His ambivalence between struggle and surrender was aggravated by a theological complication: Wouldn't he betray his religious beliefs if he gave up hope of healing? It is significant for the present context that Mr. W.'s struggles were also about different understandings of Christian hope for healing. His personal advisor advocated resolutely the hope for miraculous recovery and conducted regularly healing prayer ceremonies for Mr W. and other people. As a kind of medium, she represented all those who believe that the Christian call to healing has nothing to do with modern medicine and state-regulated healthcare, and that prayer ceremonies, prophetic inspirations, laying on of hands, anointing rituals, consecrated materials, and exorcism are the main means of divine healing (cf. Brown 2011). According to this counter-cultural options (cf. Balboni 2013),[4] Christian healing differs fundamentally from secular medicine, nursing, and psychology.

On the other side stood the chaplain. By carrying out his work as a member of the interprofessional team while being mandated by the Catholic Church, he embodied an approach described by Miroslav Volf as "internal difference". It involves an attempt "of living Christian difference within a given culture: the majority of the elements of a culture will be taken up but transformed from within" (Volf 2011, 91). On this option, the Christian call to healing is primarily met in taking shared responsibility for a holistic and just healthcare by using and transforming all available methods. The goal is to (trans-)form secular healthcare "from within" through Christian involvement in its design.

4 Balboni distinguishes three theological approaches that coincide on many points with the options outlined here.

To limit the Christian call to healing to religious practices is to misjudge its universalism epitomized by Jesus and the Good Samaritan. It would mean closing oneself off from developments in modern healthcare and failing to recognise one's share of responsibility for them. Therefore, since the early days of the CPE, Christian healthcare chaplaincy has pursued the second option. To sound the possibilities for "the internal difference", it is necessary to start out not with the biomedical paradigm, rightly criticized for his reductionism, but with a nuanced and widely accepted understanding of healthcare. If there is one document that fits this description, it is the New York *Hastings Center Report on the Goals of Medicine*, published in 1996. Fourteen groups of countries were involved in this consensus project, which was led by the renowned medical ethicist Daniel Callahan. The Hastings Center Report offers a reliable and substantively nuanced foundation for the clarification sought here. In a critical analysis of modern medicine's limitations and downsides, the report concludes that a reformulation of the current goals of medicine is necessary for economic, socio-political and clinical reasons. Four main goals of equal importance are set out:

1. *The prevention of disease and injury and the promotion and maintenance of health.* It is an ancient goal of medicine "to help people live more harmoniously with their environment, an aim that must be pursued from the beginning of life to its very end" (Callahan 1996).
2. *The relief of pain and suffering caused by maladies.* The report distinguishes physical pain from mental suffering and calls for more attention to be paid to the latter.
3. *The care and cure of those with a malady, and the care of those who cannot be cured.* The distinctions introduced in this context are especially significant for our discussion: "The healing function of medicine encompasses both curing and caring, and healing may in a broader sense be possible even in those cases where medicine cannot cure. It can heal by helping a person cope effectively with permanent maladies" (Callahan 1996, 12).
4. *The avoidance of premature death and the pursuit of a peaceful death.* As with the second goal, the report emphasises the importance of palliative care and the responsibility doctors share for "humane care of the dying" (Callahan 1996, 13). No consensus could be reached on the issues of euthanasia and assisted suicide.

It should be noted that the overemphasis on curative medicine criticised in the first part of the Report is clearly rectified in the four goals cited. Thus, *cure* does not appear as an independent goal, but in connection with the *care* of people with curable and incurable diseases. It is also emphasised here that there is a form of *healing* that lies – at least partially – outside the realm of curative medicine. Through a differentiated and open understanding of the goals of today's medicine and healthcare, the *Hastings Center Report* offers a helpful instrument for specifying the relationship between secular healthcare and the Christian call to healing. Where and how could the "Christian difference" be inscribed in the four goals of medicine?

Consider the following three options: The "Christian difference" concerns, first, the manner – or the spirit – in which people work towards the stated goals. Professional interaction with patients is shaped by basic attitudes and beliefs. To trust in God's healing presence in clinical encounters will have an impact on therapeutic processes. Second, from the perspective of Christian faith, patients are far more than recipients of help and care. Seeing them as bearer of significant stories and as a treasure hidden in fragile vessels, enriches professional relationships. Third, the Christian difference can also be realised by implement of the goals of medicine in a specific way or context. One example of this is the modern hospice movement, which has contributed to a profound change in the way we deal now with dying and death.

3 Healthcare Chaplaincy is Specialized Spiritual Care

In the 20th century, Christian nurses, doctors, and chaplains all contributed to the development of modern forms of spiritual care. Moreover, clinical social workers, psychotherapists, and other health professionals can also understand their work as an answer to the Christian call for healing. Each professional group has its own assets to bring to bear within the context of interprofessional spiritual care. The contribution of each of these professions merits closer analysis, validation, and encouragement. Healthcare chaplains are specialists in a field in which nurses, doctors and other healthcare or social professionals are primary caregivers. The distinction between generalist and specialised spiritual care helps to keep in view what is distinctive about the complementary professional approaches, while at the same time relating them to each other.

From a theological perspective, the difference between generalist and specialised spiritual care lies also in a special mandate and in the representational role of chaplains. Chaplains are spiritual intermediaries of trust. They are distinguished *ex professo* by the fact that their own situation in the field of religion and spirituality is, to a certain extent, connected to their professional role and thus must be declared. In the context of the Christian call to healing, they represent a particular faith tradition in secular health institutions. At the same time, they are contact points for religious and spiritual concerns in general.

What does it mean to be a good healthcare chaplain? Peter Sedgwick investigates this question in a discussion of chaplaincy and ethics (Sedgwick 2016). The question concerns both the professional ethics of chaplains and the quality criteria by which chaplaincy work is to be evaluated. Sedgwick contends that chaplains are responsible to a twofold ethical framework: that of the institution for which they work and that of their religious community. This twofold obligation may lead to tensions in everyday healthcare chaplaincy. The question whether and in what form spiritual care may and should be offered in a case of assisted suicide is an example of this. However, tensions between different professional obligations and between institutional and personal value systems are not unique to healthcare chaplaincy, but occur in the medical, nursing and psychotherapeutic professions as well.[5] Ethical competence therefore also involves dealing with such tensions in a reflective way.[6]

A professional ethics for healthcare chaplaincy must also include a commitment to *therapeutic* professionalism, and this leads us back to the Christian call to healing. While chaplaincy aims to do good, it may nevertheless sometimes have adverse effects. For this reason, it is subject, in clinical contexts, to professional quality standards as well as to the globally applicable principles of medical ethics, those of non-maleficence and beneficence, as well as to that of autonomy (Beauchamp and Childress 2012). This means that chaplains are not only required to carry out their work with all due diligence but have to also demonstrate that they support patients in a verifiable and effective way. It should be obvious: Chaplains must not fall short of the ethical and professional standards that apply in health institutions (Peeters 2020). The duty of therapeutic vigilance, critical self-examination and self-restraint is even more urgent because the churches have in recent decades undermined the trust placed in them through the actions of amateurish and abusive chaplains. A 2004 document of the Evangelical Church of Germany (EKD) clearly expresses this desideratum:

"It is enormously helpful for the healthcare chaplains themselves if they systematically bring the essential processes and structures of their professional and economic organisation into discussion, aligns themselves with their goals, test their character against the yardstick of these goals and dedicate themselves to continuous quality improvement on the basis of the results. In this way, it is pos-

5 Mohrmann (2008, 18–23, 20) gives the example the tension between the physician's obligation to be patient-oriented and that of training future professionals.

6 For the relationship between spiritual care and ethics counselling see the contribution of Traugott Roser in this volume.

sible to learn from experience in a sustainable and imaginative way and to shape social reality. Actions are not changed by abstractly changing mental outlooks first; rather, an attentive and careful approach can broaden mental outlooks. The initiative in this regard should lie with the healthcare chaplaincy itself" (EKD 2004, 32).

According to Margaret Moormann, healthcare chaplaincy is subject to an "ethic of accountability". Chaplains must give an account of what they do and with what objectives, of how good chaplaincy care can be assessed and how binding quality assurance is conducted (Mohrmann 2008, 20). If this is taken seriously within the framework of the standards of the healthcare sector, it has important consequences: Chaplains working in healthcare cannot simply assume that their services (and they themselves) are good for the people they are attending; this is something they must be able to demonstrate. They must also be prepared to base their actions on the current state of knowledge and to allow themselves to be guided by new evidence (Grossoehme 2020, 99f). Professional healthcare chaplaincy presupposes chaplaincy research that investigates which forms of chaplaincy care are helpful for which contexts and which are not. To give credibility to the message they are meant to embody and to meet the basic ethical principles and professional standards that apply in healthcare, trainee chaplains must familiarize themselves with empirically based models of spiritual care and learn forms of critical self-examination. The form of healthcare chaplaincy training developed during the previous century was aimed at instilling this kind of professionalism, which must now be further developed under changed circumstances. For the reasons just given, healthcare chaplaincy work will in future have to undergo a more intensive form of quality management than has so far been the case. Chaplains would do well proactively to develop the tools for this themselves. This will involve, not least, suitable documentation instruments. Since quality monitoring requires good documentation that records chaplaincy activities in a transparent fashion.[7]

4 Christian Healthcare Chaplaincy – A Spiritual Profession

The situation of healthcare chaplains working in public institutions is analogous (not equal!) to that of academic theologians. Both professions face a similar chal-

7 An alternative is to interview patients, see Snowden and Telfer (2020).

lenge: How can the demands of a secular institution brought together with a task linked to a particular faith tradition? Furthermore, both professions rely on reference disciplines and are in danger of coalescing with them. Just as chaplaincy depends on psychology, theology depends on history, philology, philosophy, etc. This book outlines a way of dealing with this tension that corresponds to Miroslav Volf's and Matthew Croasmun's theological manifesto *For the Life of the World.* They understand doing theology as a dimension of being Christian (Volf and Croasmun 2019, 115–47). This is also true for healthcare chaplaincy; seen from this perspective, it is a spiritual practice.

The spiritual character of healthcare chaplaincy has several aspects and should not be reduced to just one: a spiritual attitude and practice; a lively relationship with a faith tradition; the symbolism of the chaplain's role, and the competence to perform spiritual rituals in a clinical context.

Spiritual attitude and practice: What Christian chaplains mediate does not come from themselves. Rather, they witness to a divine presence as a reality through which they become what they are. The radical awareness of being given everything one has is itself a gift, and not something that chaplains can acquire and possess once and for all. Continually rekindled and nurtured, this awareness can become life-determining and effective in one's actions. Therefore, Christian chaplaincy presupposes a personal practice of prayer and meditation, through which the 'agents' of chaplaincy may themselves become recipients again and again. Understood in this way, the anchoring of chaplaincy in a spiritual practice is a distinguishing attribute of the profession.

Anchoring in a faith tradition: There are many reasons why a chaplain should be endorsed by a faith community. It ties healthcare chaplaincy back to the local congregations and promotes interaction between the clinical and non-clinical spheres. Moreover, it situates healthcare chaplaincy within the multifaceted church involvement in the healthcare system and enables chaplains to speak and act on behalf of a concrete faith tradition. In this way, the community is not merely officially represented, but also spiritually present. According to MacLaren, religious and spiritual traditions fulfil a formative function for healthcare chaplaincy that can be compared to that of the schools of psychotherapy. Psychotherapists, like chaplains, practise in a particular modality: "Competence in working within one's core modality is a prerequisite for practice [. . .] having no 'spiritual modality' is not an option [. . .] a chaplain is precisely someone who has been formed within a particular wisdom tradition (Jewish, Buddhist, Sikh, Humanist, and so forth), and has developed the critical skills to be able to draw upon the resources of that tradition, and to critique its weaknesses. [. . .] it is this rootedness in the spirituality of one or more concrete, historical, wisdom traditions that makes chaplains distinctive and constitutes their 'unique selling point'." (MacLaren 2021, 36).

The symbolism of the role of chaplain: Due to complex historical developments, the role of healthcare chaplains in (post-)secular institutions is not limited to representing a specific religious tradition and community; rather, they embody the connection to an ultimate horizon of meaning, to a transcendent reality. In their role, they symbolise personal access points to the "spiritual dimension", points of contact for all kinds of religious and spiritual questions, longings, and needs. They evoke the dimension of the holy: "The difference between chaplaincy and other professions (e.g. psychotherapy and psycho-oncology) lies primarily in the horizon of meaning within which each profession listens, resonates and dignifies. In virtue of its role, chaplaincy always – but not always explicitly – dignifies within the horizon of a transcendent holiness: before God and from God" (Weiher 2015, 241–48). Chaplaincy communication is determined by this horizon of meaning, even when it is not explicitly mentioned. This leads to the fourth aspect that qualifies healthcare chaplaincy as a spiritual profession.

Competence in reflective spiritual communication and ritualisation in clinical contexts: It is critical to the professional profile of chaplaincy that it be able to articulate and ritually enact the spiritual dimension at the appropriate time and in the most fitting manner. As different as the expectations people have of healthcare chaplains may be, they are likely to converge on the basic assumption that healthcare chaplains are qualified and authorised to engage in spiritual practices, to conduct a prayer or ritual or to offer counselling on religious questions, etc. Professionalism in the performance of these practices consists of several mutually interdependent competences. These are: *(1) The competence to perceive and discern:* the ability to grasp and articulate the spiritual dimension of the predicament of individuals or whole families in a differentiated and multi-layered way. *(2) Communicative and hermeneutic competences:* the ability to address spiritual burdens and resources in a differentiated way and to provide space for narrative. *(3) Ritual competencies:* familiarity with forms of prayer, rituals, spiritual communication etc.[8] Accustomed rituals and personally acquired forms of prayer enable spontaneous action in critical situations.

In the case of Mr. W., who struggled both with God and his spiritual accompanists, all the aspects just mentioned came together. He welcomed the healthcare chaplain that supported him in his spiritual needs (prayer and Holy Communion) and served as a consultant in his questioning about the will of God, as well

8 According to Meyer-Blanck (2019, 55), "learning to pray publicly" is a characteristic of pastoral education.

as a mediator between him and the medical team. It is worth mentioning that in the four meetings with Mr. W. the chaplain was not only a caregiver but also in the position of a recipient. Even more than being a witness himself, he was the addressee of life testimony. The encounter with Mr W. had a spiritual character and enlarged his awareness about the many ways of responding to the Christian call to healing.[9]

References

Balboni, Michael J. 2013. 'A Theological Assessment of Spiritual Assessments'. *Christian Bioethics: Non-Ecumenical Studies in Medical Morality* 19 (3): 313–31. https://doi.org/10.1093/cb/cbt023.

Beauchamp, Tom L., and James F. Childress. 2012. *Principles of Biomedical Ethics*. 7th ed. New York, Oxford: Oxford University Press.

Brown, Candy Gunther. 2011. *Global Pentecostal and Charismatic Healing*. Oxford, New York: Oxford University Press.

Callahan, Daniel. 1996. 'The Goals of Medicine-Setting New Priorities'. *Hastings Center Report* 26 (6).

EKD. 2004. 'Die Kraft zum Menschsein Stärken: Leitlinien für die Evangelische Krankenhausseelsorge — Eine Orientierungshilfe'. Evangelische Kirche in Deutschland.

Grossoehme, Daniel H. 2020. 'The Role of Science in Enhancing Spiritual Care Practice'. In *Chaplaincy and the Soul of Health and Social Care*, edited by Ewan Kelly and John Swinton, 93–102. London and Philadelphia: Jessica Kingsley Publishers.

Jobin, Guy. 2020. *Spirituality in the Biomedical World: Moving between Order and "Subversion"*. Berlin: De Gruyter. https://doi.org/10.1515/9783110638950.

MacLaren, Duncan. 2021. 'All Things to All People? The Integrity of Spiritual Care in a Plural Health Service.' *Health & Social Care Chaplaincy* 9 (1): 27–41.

Meyer-Blanck, Michael. 2019. *Das Gebet*. Tübingen: Mohr Siebeck.

Mohrmann, Margaret E. 2008. 'Ethical Grounding for a Profession of Hospital Chaplaincy'. *The Hastings Center Report* 38 (6): 18–23.

Peeters, Evelyn J H. 2020. 'Quality Pastoral Relationships in Healthcare Settings: Guidelines for Codes of Ethics'. *The Journal of Pastoral Care & Counseling* 74 (1): 42–52. https://doi.org/10.1177/1542305019897555.

Peng-Keller, Simon. 2024. *Healthcare Chaplaincy as Specialised Spiritual Care – The Christian Call for Healing in a Global Health Context*. Translated by David Dolby. 1st ed. Göttingen: Vandenhoeck & Ruprecht.

Peng-Keller, Simon, and David Neuhold, eds. 2020. *Charting Spiritual Care: The Emerging Role of Chaplaincy Records in Global Health Care*. Cham: Springer International Publishing. https://doi.org/10.1007/978-3-030-47070-8.

9 With the words of Traugott Roser (this volume), I could say, that the encounter with Mr W. "affected my personal beliefs, spirituality, and existence, both challenging and making me grow."

Sedgwick, Peter. 2016. 'Chaplaincy and Ethics: What Does It Mean to Be a Good Chaplain?' In *A Handbook of Chaplaincy Studies. Understanding Spiritual Care in Public Places*, edited by Chris Swift, Mark Cobb, and Andrew Todd, 97–108. London: Routledge.

Snowden, Austyn, and Iain Telfer. 2020. 'The Story of the Scottish Patient Reported Outcome Measure'. In *Chaplaincy and the Soul of Health and Social Care*, edited by Ewan Kelly and John Swinton, 187–201. London and Philadelphia: Jessica Kingsley Publishers.

Theißen, Gerd. 2008. 'Symbolisches Heilen in der Nachfolge Jesu. Neutestamentliche Überlegungen zum Diakonischen Heilungsauftrag'. In *Diakonie und Bildung*, edited by Johannes Eurich and Christian Oelschlägel, 43–67. Stuttgart: Kohlhammer.

Volf, Miroslav. 2011. *A Public Faith: How Followers of Christ Should Serve the Common Good*. Grand Rapids, MI: Brazos Press.

Volf, Miroslav, and Matthew Croasmun. 2019. *For the Life of the World: Theology That Makes a Difference*. Grand Rapids: Brazos Press.

WCC. 2017. '"Our Calling to Health and Healing Is as Strong as Ever"'. World Council of Churches. 25 May 2017. https://www.oikoumene.org/news/our-calling-to-health-and-healing-is-as-strong-as-ever.

Weiher, Erhard. 2015. 'Seelsorge – das machen doch alle!?: Kompetenzen und Grenzen in Spiritual Care'. *Diakonia* 46:241–48.

Anne Vandenhoeck

Authenticity and the Metaphor of the Chameleon. On the Importance of Spiritual Identity in Healthcare Chaplaincy

Abstract: More and more people in Western societies do not identify with organized religions or belief systems. Should chaplains follow suit? And should those with a spiritual tradition hide it to become chameleons, adapting to the spirituality of those in front of them? There is a fluidity and universality in spiritual care. A comparison made by MacLaren (2021) states there are common characteristics in therapy. However, therapists have schools, and chaplains should have a spiritual identity tied to a spiritual tradition. There is no such thing as neutrality, chaplains need their spiritual self to do spiritual care. In this contribution, I advocate for spiritual caregivers' rootedness in spiritual traditions in the midst of ongoing processes of secularization, pluralization, and detraditionalization. How can chaplains be authentic in spiritual care for patients against the background of a decreased value of a spiritual identity based on a spiritual tradition? An exploration of integrity and authenticity is needed to understand the communication about identity in spiritual caregiving. There is great variety in the prominence of the spiritual identity of the chaplain in relation to the patient. However, it is of importance to the quality of spiritual care. Creating space for the patient's spirituality requires expert handling of one's own spiritual identity without denying it.

1 Introduction

When I worked for a year as a chaplain in a hospital in the USA, I befriended the rabbi in the team. He generously invited me to a synagogue, a Yom Kippur service and so on. One day, he told me the following story. In his previous position in a different hospital, he was the head of the spiritual care service, which also had a Catholic priest. After a particularly tough week in the hospital, where the priest rarely saw his bed due to the many calls for the last sacrament, he received the priest in his office. The priest was so exhausted that he put the vessel with ointment on the rabbi's desk and said: 'I can't stay here for another minute. I need to recover physically, emotionally and spiritually. I called priests in parishes, but no one could take over. If there is a call, you will need to go.' The rabbi stared at the

https://doi.org/10.1515/9783112205839-003

vessel with disbelief and terror. Lo and behold, a call came. An Italian family needed a priest to visit their dying father. The rabbi went to the family and said: "I am the rabbi. My colleague, the priest, is not in the hospital now, but he gave me this vessel with very precious ointment. If you want, I can bless your father with this ointment and pray for him, as we share the same God." The family agreed, and they prayed, and the rabbi blessed the dying family member.

You could look at this case from different perspectives. A legalistic perspective would only see the fact that this was not, nor could ever count as a sacrament. A theological perspective would discuss the mediated space for God's grace. From the patient's and the family's perspective, the rabbi came when they needed support and engaged with them at a crucial point in their lives. An interfaith perspective would highlight the rabbi's emphasis on his own identity, what both traditions have in common, and what the boundaries are of his contribution. He did not pretend that he could give a sacrament nor let his identity at the door. In his authenticity and because of his openness, he was able to care spiritually for the family.

I once presented a paper on spiritual caregivers and palliative care at the network meeting of palliative care of the university and university hospital KU Leuven in Belgium. I explained that spiritual caregivers are specialists from different traditions such as Christianity, Islam, Judaism, Humanism, etc. One question from someone in the audience touched upon the subject of this reflection: 'Is a spiritual caregiver from a specific tradition still relevant, as most people do not belong to a tradition anymore?' I would like to describe and elaborate on my answer in this contribution. I told the audience member that tradition is still very relevant, not because of statistics (namely, the number of people identifying as Christians, Muslims, Humanists, Jews, and so on) but because of the goals, quality, integrity, and authenticity of spiritual care. I do believe being rooted in tradition makes a difference for spiritual care. The point I am highlighting in what follows is that being rooted in a spiritual tradition enhances the quality of spiritual care, and that spiritual caregivers can be chameleons to a certain degree – but not in the way the metaphor usually evokes in discussions. I will focus on those healthcare chaplains rooted in the Christian tradition.[1]

---

1 'Chaplain' is a word coming out of the Christian tradition and originally refers to a priest appointed to a chapel. It became a word used in the English language to refer to those doing pastoral care in different settings such as prison, hospital and army. In some parts of the world the term is adopted by other traditions and thus there are Muslim chaplains, Humanist chaplains, Jewish chaplains and so on. There is some critique about the use of the word chaplain coming from none-Christian traditions. Spiritual caregiver is a name coming out of the field of healthcare where spiritual care, spirituality, spiritual care team, generalist and specialist spiritual care are

2 The Influence of Society on Christian Healthcare Chaplaincy

As widely researched and analysed, European countries are amidst processes of secularization, detraditionalization and pluralization. Detraditionalization refers to younger generations who grew up in Christian families, received sacraments, or went to Christian schools but do not identify much with the tradition. They appreciate what they consider 'Christian values', but their knowledge of Christianity or their going to church and living faith has diminished significantly. Most people in younger generations become ever further removed from the tradition. Pluralization means that different or new faiths and beliefs enter European societies through migration and globalization. Although it seems abundantly clear what secularization is, it remains important to stress that secularization always happens within a particular culture. Every country goes through its own process of secularization, which is closely connected with its (religious) history.

Take, for example, Belgium and The Netherlands. Although we speak the same language and are neighbouring countries, our secularization process differs. The secularization process in Flanders, the Dutch-speaking part of Belgium, can be labelled as monolithic (MacLaren 2021) and is comparable to a certain degree to the way this process is taking place in France. The form of secularization in France is called *laïcité*. It can be described as pursuing a neutral public space (concerning religion and faith) in which universal citizenship is promoted (Lizotte 2020). In both Belgium and France, the Catholic Church – as the dominant and largest religion – had an influence on the entire society. The Church was omnipresent from the cradle to the grave. In a reaction against the almost absolute power of the Catholic Church in the past and due to a current fear of Islam, the secularization process today is based on a sharp rejection of the presence of religion and faith in public space. The aim is for the public to be a neutral space with regard to religious or belief persuasion. Belief or faith belongs strictly to the private sphere. It hardly needs to be demonstrated that this leads to predictable tensions, such as those around the so-called 'headscarf debate' in which wearing a headscarf in public institutions, such as state education and services, has been challenged. But this neutrality is essentially an illusion. No one is neutral, as everyone has a view of the world and life in it, whether or not shaped in part by elements of major faith traditions. In such debates, however, different interpreta-

---

common language. Spiritual caregivers refers to those healthcare professionals who are trained and hired to address the spiritual needs and resources of patients and who come from various faiths and beliefs systems.

tions of the concept of neutrality are used. Take the example of the debate about whether or not a civil servant can wear a headscarf. Those in favour of a neutral public space include in neutrality the appearance of civil servants (no reference to a religion or belief should be visible), while opponents point to the diversity in society and emphasize that it is not the appearance of civil servants that should be neutral, but that their service should be exercised neutrally (in the same qualitative and efficient manner as by every civil servant).

The process of secularization in The Netherlands evolves differently. Through its history of trade and colonization, the Netherlands has been a country with different faiths and beliefs. Mainly Protestant and Catholic traditions at first, but gradually, more and more different religions. Secularization in The Netherlands embraces the existence of different religions and beliefs and does not strive to have a neutral public space, although, of course, secularization always implies that religions and beliefs are no longer the centre of society and the main perspective on daily life. There is, however, less hostility towards religious traditions and belief systems in public spaces.

These different processes of secularization also had an impact on the way chaplaincy is organized. In Belgium, specifically in the Flemish-speaking part, there is only one professional association for healthcare chaplains: the Catholic one (around 200 members). Healthcare chaplains from other backgrounds are scarcer: around 40 Humanist chaplains are working in the Flemish part of Belgium, around five Protestant chaplains and five Muslim chaplains. They are not organized in professional associations. The French-speaking part of Belgium has fewer professional chaplains and works more with volunteers. The Catholic professional association inevitably leads the dialogue among the different faiths in political lobbying and professional development. The different faiths have agreed upon a generic name for all chaplains in healthcare: “spiritual caregivers” (spiritueel zorgverleners). That does not mean that spiritual caregivers do not have the ethical duty to tell patients their own faith background. Patients have a right to know. In The Netherlands, there is one professional association with several subdivisions: the Catholic, Protestant, Humanist, Pandit, Jewish, Buddhist, Orthodox, and the subdivision of unaffiliated chaplains, those not representing a faith or belief.

3 Spiritual Caregivers as ‘Chameleons’

Christian spiritual caregivers also visit patients who do not identify with the Christian tradition or any other tradition. Still, they provide spiritual care for them. Does that make them chameleons—co-colouring with whatever the patient believes? When you go to a funeral in Belgium which occurs in a funeral home, one of the undertakers usually leads the service. Those services are based on the preferences expressed by the deceased's family. The undertaker takes the role of the 'neutral' presider: they read the texts (religious or secular) chosen by the family, performs prayers if asked, and lead the symbolic acts of the ceremony. The spiritual identity of the undertaker is not known, and that is precisely the intention. They wear a different hat, symbolically speaking, for each funeral service.

In this realm, some mention the metaphor of the spiritual caregiver as a 'chameleon' (Kruizinga 2022; Vandenhoeck 2022; Braam 2022). The chameleon metaphor usually evokes the image of an animal that changes colour to blend in with the surroundings. If the background is red, the chameleon turns red. To give a more extreme example: if a humanist spiritual caregiver visits a Christian patient and the patient wants a prayer, often without knowing the background of the spiritual caregiver, the humanist spiritual caregiver, who is not a believer, will pray with the patient. In this view of spiritual care, the spiritual caregiver's spiritual identity does not matter much. Anke Liefbroer researched the involvement of the tradition/spirituality of the spiritual caregiver and distinguished between a specialist-particularist perspective and a specialist-universalist perspective (Liefbroer et al. 2017; Liefbroer and Nagel 2021). In the particularist perspective, where spirituality is seen as a domain of specialists or experts, the spirituality/tradition of the spiritual caregiver is deemed important. From the universalist perspective, spirituality is also seen as the domain of experts, but the spirituality/tradition of the spiritual caregiver is not important. I do think the spirituality of the spiritual caregiver matters in relation to the patient. The question is then if there is a way that values the spiritual caregiver's spiritual tradition but also allows for the more universalist and perhaps fluid elements of spiritual care. Some Catholic chaplains, for example, will perform a ritual for a patient where God may not be mentioned. These Catholic chaplains motivate their decision from a diaconal perspective: serving those in spiritual need in God's name. Though his name remains unmentioned, it is deeply present in the motivation of the Catholic chaplain to perform the ritual to help people grieve or say farewell. This motivation leads to an affirmation of identity rather than denying it.

Yet, all of the above raises questions about authenticity and integrity. The image of the chameleon is used to describe the spiritual caregiver in a highly diversified faith landscape. When threatened by the enemy, chameleons indeed change colour (and patterns in that colour) to adapt to or blend into the environment (co-colouring). However, that is not the only reason. Chameleons also use colour and pattern to give social signals to members of their species about their own emotions. So, in addition to co-colouring, there is also communication about identity. The analogy of the chameleon is simplified in the chaplaincy discussion and in its current association, and is less appropriate to describe the balancing exercises between the identity of the spiritual caregiver and the context of diversity. An exploration of integrity and authenticity is needed to understand the communication about identity in spiritual caregiving.

The concept of integrity takes on different nuances depending on the context. For example, integrity is defined as an attitude within a professional context in which a person adheres to a moral or ethical code. Other nuances emerge when integrity is described as consistency. A person of integrity acts consistently based on how they present themselves and the ideals they pursue. Annelieke Damen and others similarly describe integrity in relation to professionalism (Damen et al. 2020). They advocate integrity in researching the outcomes of spiritual care. This includes taking into account the specificity of the profession of spiritual caregivers and spiritual care. Integrity is a coveted social good. Integrous individuals are seen as trustworthy and honest. The difference between integrity and authenticity is not always clear. Authenticity is usually seen as a higher and personal form of integrity. Authenticity, then, is no longer just acting consistently according to ethical and moral codes or stated ideals. Those codes or ideals are also an expression of your deepest values, beliefs and commitments. In authenticity, there is a deep identification with codes or ideals. Integrity and authenticity do not always go together. To be authentic, you sometimes have to go against prevailing codes. Authenticity can create social ripples because someone goes against conventions and norms. You can also have integrity in following a code or ideal at all costs but lose authenticity.

Both integrity and authenticity strike me as particularly important for spiritual caregivers, especially when engaging in dialogue with an ever-changing reality of faiths and beliefs. Integrity can be connected to spiritual care in several ways. It seems fundamental that integrity begins with responding to the patient's right to know the spiritual caregiver's religious or personal beliefs. In other words, it remains essential that spiritual caregivers also present themselves from the tradition to which they confess. And if it is an unaffiliated spiritual caregiver, there should be at least openness about their lack of affiliation. Authenticity is the point of departure from which the spiritual caregivers want to act with integrity around their own faith or belief. In that sense, I do not think that the spiritual caregiver who does not believe in God and prays with the patient without communicating this fact is authentic.

Some researchers stress the necessity of being grounded in a specific tradition, having respect for the religious/spiritual identity of the patient and showing an openness about one's own faith tradition (MacLaren 2021). The (well-developed) specific spirituality of the chaplain can also be used as a touchstone, a mirror, a breaking point, a challenge, or an inspiration to a patient. Chaplains are trained to work with their spirituality as well as with that of the patient. Another argument is that being a representative of a faith tradition guarantees quality, a tested spirituality and not representing only one's own spirituality. Faith or belief organizations offer their chaplains continuing education, which guarantees quality. The spiritual traditions incorporated in faith and belief systems also offer common traditions and practices, and wisdom towards challenges in spiritual development. Chaplains thus receive tools, insights, inspiration and confrontation for their spiritual identity from spiritual traditions.

4 Christian Spiritual Care within Pluralistic Healthcare Settings

MacLaren, head of the spiritual and bereavement care service at the National Health Service (NHS) in Scotland, highlights the importance of integrity for spiritual care in a spiritually diverse healthcare context in a contribution to the *Journal of Health and Social Care Chaplaincy*. He reflects on how the organization of spiritual care has adapted because of the spiritually plural landscape in the UK, as well as because of the professionalization (MacLaren 2021). The comparison between Flanders and the Netherlands on the one hand and Scotland and England on the other is compelling. Even in the latter two countries, there are differences in the way in which they respond to pluralism and secularization. MacLaren's question is whether the possibility of integrity and authenticity are sufficiently safeguarded in either response.

In England, comparable to The Netherlands, the diversity of religions and faiths has been embraced and translated into the composition of teams of spiritual caregivers who are a mix of the various local spiritual traditions (plural secularization). An Anglican priest, a Catholic lay pastor, a Muslim consultant and a pagan consultant, for example, may work together in one team. This gives the impression that only patients of those spiritual traditions can find support, whereas, in practice, most spiritual care providers go to anyone in need. So, according to MacLaren, the downside of this model is that not all patients have representatives of their spiritual tradition and access to spiritual care. And what about patients who do not identify with a particular tradition?

In Scotland, they have created a neutral space for spiritual care through generic spiritual caregivers (monolithic secularization). They leave their spiritual identity at the front door of the hospital, so to speak, and become a "neutral" agent. In theory, this would mean that an outside priest or pastor should come in when a patient desires a religious ritual. The daily practice runs more smoothly: spiritual care remains intertwined with religious care when patients desire it. Yet in this model, the identity of the spiritual caregiver is minimized in favour of a "neutral" space for spiritual care. The drawback is that suppressing one's own spiritual roots strains the integrity and authenticity of the spiritual caregiver (MacLaren 2021).

MacLaren sees, in addition to multi-faith teams and generic spiritual care providers, a third avenue for organizing spiritual care in a spiritually diverse healthcare context. This third path connects the spiritual caregiver's spiritual identity and access to spiritual care for all. The middle way, then, starts from the link between the spiritual caregiver's spiritual identity and the competencies they possess, such as being able to use one's own spirituality to recognize elements of the patient's spirituality. Thus, spiritual caregivers do not need to leave their spirituality behind. They need their spiritual self to do the job: "Spiritual caregivers have professionally reflected deeply on a range of themes relevant to spiritual care, using perspectives from specific spiritual and theological traditions" (MacLaren 2021, 33).

To substantiate this third way, MacLaren (2021) draws on the comparison with psychologists or therapists who are, without exception, formed within certain schools (behavioural therapy, cognitive therapy, etc.). Being trained within a school means being able to draw on the resources within that tradition and being critical of it. The particularity of the therapist does not prevent therapy from being supportive for many because there are also universalistic factors determining the support therapy can offer – such as the quality of the care relationship. For MacLaren, the way therapists deal with their school is an inspiration for spiritual caregivers. He crystallizes that into three points for spiritual caregivers: 1. Having no "school" is not an option. Spiritual caregivers need to be rooted in a spiritual tradition. A set of generic skills is not enough. Moreover, those roots need to be nurtured permanently. 2. In spiritual care, there is also a field shared by all faiths and beliefs. After all, spiritual care, from whatever particularity, always touches on core values, ethical frames of reference, spiritual traditions, lore of texts, etc. From there, a common language about spiritual care can emerge. 3. Therapists do not constantly push their particularity in clients' faces. They are open about the school to which they belong but do not bring it up at random. The needs and questions of patients should come first for spiritual caregivers. One can work from a strong sense of identity and yet not have to constantly formulate it. Here MacLaren uses the expression "invisible roots" (MacLaren 2021, 37): the roots do not have to be visible all the time, but they are there and need to be nurtured.

In his contribution, MacLaren looks for space for the patient, whatever their spiritual needs and resources, in which spiritual care can take place in dialogue with a spiritual caregiver who is rooted in a spiritual tradition. Creating space for the patient's spirituality requires professional handling of one's own spiritual identity without denying it. Not denying one's own spiritual identity contributes to a greater space for integrity and authenticity.

5 Christian Spiritual Care

Being rooted in Christian tradition and spirituality is important for Christian spiritual caregivers, as is *diakonia*. The service to others is at the heart of the Church. Healthcare, from a Christian perspective, has always been diaconal. When society did not care for mental health patients, for example, Catholic congregations stepped in and made it their mission to set up mental health hospitals. Before enumerating the mutual enrichment between *diakonia* and identity, I would like to explain the formal aspect of being a Christian chaplain in a mental health, general or university hospital or nursing home in Belgium. How does a healthcare institution hire a chaplain? And what is the role of the faith community?

Catholic chaplains in Belgium are hired and remunerated by hospitals or nursing homes and sent by the Church. This means that, in the best possible scenario, the vicar for Caritas in the Catholic Church is consulted about the job description for the vacancy, is involved in the interviews with candidates and has to agree with the selected candidate. In Flanders, one speaks of spiritual caregivers' double bond or loyalty: to the healthcare facility and the sending faith community or belief system. This bond with the sending faith community presupposes from the chaplain a loyalty towards this spiritual tradition and a willingness to form oneself permanently within the range of this tradition. On the part of the faith community, this bond presupposes an offer of intervision, guidance, formation, and supervision. Regarding quality assurance of spiritual care, the main providers are the faith communities, the training institutes (in dioceses and Catholic colleges and universities) and the Professional Association for Catholic Healthcare Chaplains. Unfortunately, there is no formal or legal agreement between the Church and the hospitals or nursing homes regarding their involvement in hiring new healthcare chaplains. This process of involving the Catholic Church is based on a "gentlemen's agreement" dating from the time when religion was evidently present in healthcare and culture. In today's society, healthcare facilities honour this gentlemen's agreement progressively lesser. With advancing secularization and detraditionalization, the double bond is thus under pressure. Directors and managers increasingly ask themselves why the dioceses must be involved, as the healthcare institution pays for the chaplain. The dioceses are generally more concerned about parish communities than about spiritual care in health care. Chaplains themselves are not always happy representing the institute of the church and experience pressure on their loyalty.

Some directors and managers take the first step in hiring unaffiliated spiritual caregivers because they think they represent all patients who no longer identify with a religion or faith tradition. However, this group of spiritual caregivers does not have access to any existing specific training for this profession. They are usually nurses, psychologists or social workers interested in spiritual care who, at best, have taken a course or module in spiritual care. Needless to say, there is hardly any quality assurance for this group of spiritual caregivers.

6 The Role of the Christian Spiritual Caregiver in Interprofessional Spiritual Care

Interprofessional spiritual care is on the rise in literature, training and research. It refers to the perspective that all healthcare professionals need to integrate care for the patient's spirituality. This aspect of care needs to be present in team meetings and in electronic patient files. In order to establish interprofessional spiritual care, training and education of healthcare professionals in generalist spiritual care is required. Generalist spiritual care is different from specialist spiritual care, meaning a healthcare professional does not need to have the experience; knowledge and training a chaplain has. Interprofessional spiritual care explicitly includes the presence of specialist spiritual care. The chaplain is part of the team and takes the role of the specialist in spiritual care. A good practice is a small project at Mayo Clinic, Florida, for outpatients with brain tumours.[2] The chaplain, taught the social worker, who meets every outpatient, to screen for spiritual distress using the FICA tool (Borneman, Ferrell, and Puchalski 2010). When patients do have spiritual distress, the social worker refers them to the chaplain. At the same time, nurses and physicians are trained by the chaplain in basic attention to spiritual care with the aim of integrating it more into whole-person care in the outpatient clinic. This illustrates the chaplain's role in interprofessional spiritual care and in the team's whole-person care.

2 See the 2022 Spirituality & Health Demonstration Project based at the George Washington Institute for Spirituality (GWish).

The role of the Christian spiritual caregiver in interprofessional spiritual care is threefold. First, the Christian spiritual caregiver is an expert in the Christian tradition. That expertise is valid when, for example, end-of-life care is discussed with a Christian patient. In many cases, the spiritual caregiver also has more knowledge of different religious or belief traditions than other healthcare professionals. Spiritual caregivers, in any case, through their insider perspective, have more of a general feeling about what might be essential to discuss with patients from the point of view of their spirituality. They will also connect patients or family members to representatives of their faith or belief when needed. A second role is being who they are: Christian chaplains doing pastoral and spiritual care. They are conscious of their identity and the role it plays. They can handle their own spirituality in a professional manner and are aware they react from a Christian frame of reference. They display integrity and authenticity as they are not neutral spiritual givers but act from a place of dialogue. A third role Christian spiritual caregivers have is to advocate for spiritual care: connecting with leadership, integrating spiritual care on all levels, training other healthcare professionals, doing research or being research literate . . . In the case of Christian healthcare institutions, the role of Christian spiritual caregivers is integral to the culture and identity to which they contribute.

7 Conclusion

This contribution has advocated for the chaplain's spiritual rootedness, tied to authenticity and integrity in relation to a patient's spirituality. In that regard, I would like to conclude with a personal reflection on authenticity and identity. I was born a Catholic in a Catholic country that started the process of secularization in the late fifties, well before I was born. Why did I remain in my faith and tradition when so many of my generation did not? I believe it had to do with the family I was raised in, where faith was about warmth and love. It certainly had to do with the parish we lived in, where faith was joyful and needed to be celebrated. The schools I went to were run by religious sisters who showed me how women can contribute to church and society and make a difference. I had Jesuit mentors who showed me that faith and intellect can go together seamlessly. But most of all, I felt called by God.

Because of the secularization in my country, I am used to meeting surprise, curiosity, or even hostility regarding the spiritual choices I made in different phases of life: to remain in the faith I was born, to study theology, to become a chaplain, to do research in chaplaincy, to teach theology, to preside over rituals.

The reactions never get old, but my attitude towards them has changed. When I was in my twenties, I experienced it as mortifying to say I studied theology and became a chaplain. I was ashamed because it was not a popular choice, and I had many conversations with friendly people on trains or planes who asked me what I did. I dreaded those questions and never told the whole truth, just that I was working with people dying in hospitals, which always got a very positive response. I wanted to shield myself from hostility and protect the most valuable part of my being against continuous criticism.

Times have changed. In our society today, people additionally feel hostility towards the Catholic Church because of its past, where some clergy abused the faithful. At the university, I need to deal with a very absolute perspective on the power of science and the view that religion is the opposite of knowledge. And I have changed, too. I am more comfortable in sharing my spiritual identity because I realized as I grew older that no one has the power to take away my deepest beliefs or my relationship with God. I discovered how Catholic I was when working abroad in multifaith teams of chaplains. Things I never realized or took for granted, as normal as breathing, suddenly defined me as Catholic. And finally, chaplaincy and teaching have taught me to be seen as a representative of a faith tradition, the good, and the bad and everything in between.

I am a Christian chaplain, open to people who want me to make time and space for their questions, rituals, and other spiritual needs. I experienced that my own faith can be an enrichment and inspiration to them, a means to grow in spirituality, a mirror for their own hardships in life, or just a topic of conversation and sometimes a cause for criticism. And that is how it should be. I have never and will never foist my faith upon people. Being a Christian chaplain is a balancing act between your spiritual identity and that of others. My perspective is that of seeing God in the person in front of me. That person may not see the same thing, and that is fine. But it is my motivation to engage with those who are on my path.

I believe that the future of Christian chaplaincy is tied to authenticity in spiritual identity, lived spirituality, integration into healthcare cultures, increased professionalism, and openness to everyone's spirituality.

References

Borneman, Tami, Betty Ferrell, and Christina M Puchalski. 2010. 'Evaluation of the FICA Tool for Spiritual Assessment'. Journal of Pain and Symptom Management 40 (2): 163–73.

Braam, Arjan W. 2022. 'De Kameleon: Welke Kleuren?' In Van Alle Markten Thuis? Levensbeschouwelijke Diversiteit in de Zorg Voor Zin, edited by Kees De Groot and Anne Vandenhoeck, 97: 55–60. Tilburg, Netherlands: KSGV.

Damen, Annelieke, Carmen Schumann, Carlo Leget, and George Fitchett. 2020. 'Can Outcome Research Respect the Integrity of Chaplaincy? A Review of Outcome Studies'. Journal of Health Care Chaplaincy 26 (4): 131–58. https://doi.org/10.1080/08854726.2019.1599258.

Kruizinga, Renske. 2022. 'De Unieke En Veelkleurige Praktijk van Interlevensbeschouwelijke Geestelijke Verzorging'. In Van Alle Markten Thuis? Levensbeschouwelijke Diversiteit in de Zorg Voor Zin, edited by Kees De Groot and Anne Vandenhoeck, 97:15–34. Tilburg, Netherlands: KSVG.

Liefbroer, Anke I, and Ineke Nagel. 2021. 'Does Faith Concordance Matter? A Comparison of Clients' Perceptions in Same versus Interfaith Spiritual Care Encounters with Chaplains in Hospitals'. Pastoral Psychology 70 (4): 349–77.

Liefbroer, Anke I, Erik Olsman, R Ruard Ganzevoort, and Faridi S van Etten-Jamaludin. 2017. 'Interfaith Spiritual Care: A Systematic Review'. Journal of Religion and Health 56 (5): 1776–93. https://doi.org/10.1007/s10943-017-0369-1.

Lizotte, Christopher. 2020. 'Laïcité as Assimilation, Laïcité as Negotiation: Political Geographies of Secularism in the French Public School'. Political Geography 77 (March):102121. https://doi.org/10.1016/j.polgeo.2019.102121.

MacLaren, Duncan. 2021. 'All Things to All People? The Integrity of Spiritual Care in a Plural Health Service.' Health & Social Care Chaplaincy 9 (1): 27–41.

Vandenhoeck, Anne. 2022. 'Spirituele Zorgverleners En Spirituele Zorg. Een Vlaams Perspectief Op Levensbeschouwelijke Diversiteit'. In Van Alle Markten Thuis? Levensbeschouwelijke Diversiteit in de Zorg Voor Zin, edited by Kees De Groot and Anne Vandenhoeck, 97:15–34. Tilburg, Netherlands: KSGV.

Tracy Balboni, Michael Balboni

"Your Faith has Made You Well". Christian Healthcare Chaplaincy and Goals of Christian Healing

Abstract: Christian healthcare chaplaincy is founded on Christ himself – his life, teachings, and healings as well as his death and resurrection. His repeated words spoken in the context of his healings, "Your faith has made you well", provide a framework for Christian spiritual care and the goals of Christian healing. These words embody the source of healing, the process by which healing takes place, and the goal to which Christian healing is directed. Employing theological reflection and a patient case, this chapter aims to illuminate this Christ-centered framework and illustrate how it informs Christian spiritual care in the medical setting. Accordingly, Christian healthcare chaplaincy is sourced in faith in the triune God, centered on personal and communal practices of restoring wholeness and directed to ultimate wholeness found in Christ.

1 Introduction

"Your faith has made you well." These words of Jesus are thrice repeated in the Gospels in the context of miraculous healings (Matthew 9:22, Mark 10:52, and Luke 17:19). Depending on translation, this statement is rendered as faith has "made you whole" or "healed you." Though at first glance a simple statement, these repeated words of Jesus encompass the source, mode and goals of Christian healing. In this way, they form a key to unlock a Christian response to Jesus' calling to "heal the sick." Christian healthcare chaplains, together with other Christian clinicians, are hence called upon to consider this central proclamation by Jesus as a foundational piece to the practice of spiritual care.

This chapter is a meditation and theological reflection on these words of Christ, together with other related scriptures informing the practice of Christian health and healing. We recognize other alternative theological reflections, both from within and outside the Christian tradition, both humanistic and from within other religions, which are important to consider. This chapter is an example of a tradition-mediated approach toward spiritual care, which was highlighted in *Hostility to Hospitality* (Tracy Balboni and Balboni 2018), a book-length argument that identified why spiritual care should be approached from within particular spiri-

https://doi.org/10.1515/9783112205839-004

tual traditions. Even as this volume considers a common future vision for "Christian" healthcare chaplaincy, it necessitates re-engagement with the original sources and teachings of Christ (*ad fontes*). It is upon considering the implications of the words and teachings of Jesus, that the shaping of spiritual care and chaplaincy moves toward a self-consciously "Christian" identity. Additionally, this meditation will be set within the context of a patient case, both to illustrate the source, mode, and goals of Christian healing and to equip the reader with practical examples of how a theology of Christian spiritual care might be applied in practice. Finally, we briefly consider how these spiritual goals fit within the extant structures of healthcare, and how Christian spiritual caregivers can, responding to this foundational calling, provide Christ's healing to the larger healthcare context.

2 Case of Ms. James

Carol James (pseudonyms are used throughout) is a 64-year-old woman – a non-smoker – who 2.5 years prior to presentation was diagnosed with widely metastatic non-small cell lung cancer. She has had an excellent response to her systemic therapies, as well as multiple courses of stereotactic radiosurgery for brain metastases. Within the past few months, however, she has had disease progression despite a recent switch in her systemic therapy. She recently enrolled on a phase I trial, for which she is awaiting therapy initiation. During this time, she rapidly develops debilitating fatigue and anorexia. She also develops worsening shortness of breath, fever and cough, prompting her husband, John James, to bring her to the emergency department (ED). On evaluation, Carol has cancer-related cachexia and medical work-up demonstrates masses encasing the trachea and bilateral mainstem bronchi with severe narrowing, right greater than left. She also has post-obstructive pneumonia on the right, with associated partial lung collapse. Imaging shows diffuse progression in her liver metastases, with associated liver dysfunction evidenced in her elevated liver enzymes. Her oxygen requirement increases over the course of her ED stay, and ultimately, she is intubated and admitted to the intensive care unit (ICU). She requires ventilator and presser support in additional to broad spectrum antibiotics. Thoracic surgery performs a bronchoscopy, noting narrowing of the airways at the carina and bilateral mainstem bronchi – a stent could not be deployed. The ICU team discusses with John having radiation oncology see Ms. James for urgent initiation of radiation therapy to her thoracic disease. The radiation oncology team is called to see the patient in emergent consultation.

Upon arrival at her bedside in the ICU, Carol is sedated and intubated. John is at her side using a damp towel to gently wipe her face. After Daniel, the radiation oncologist, introduces himself, John looks relieved, saying, "I'm so glad you are here. When can we get radiation started? Her cancer disappeared from her brain with her last radiation. That was a miracle we prayed for, and I just know that a miracle can happen again."

3 The Source of Christian Spiritual Care

Spiritual care of any sort – whether Christian or humanist spiritual care or otherwise – must rest on a source. To illustrate this principle in tangible terms, consider medical care of the body, termed herein as 'physical care'. The source of physical care – its energy and structures – is found within the biomedical community and its shared, communal practice of the biomedical model. This biomedical model includes shared knowledge of biological processes of health and illness and shared practices of techniques and technologies to intervene upon biological processes, such as the administration of antibiotics or robotic-assisted surgeries. Critical to recognize is that this source is grounded within a community – the shared life of a body of persons committed to biomedical knowledge and practices. Hence, the source of physical care – what comprises its underlying energy and structures – is the shared life, knowledge, and practices of the biomedical community.

Having considered the source of physical care, let us turn to the source of spiritual care. Whereas the goal of physical care is the health of the body, the goal of spiritual care is the health of the human spirit. And though the aims of physical and spiritual care are distinct from one another (albeit connected), in physical care and spiritual care there similarly must be a source of communally held energy and structures to undergird its practice. Spiritual care is hence sourced in a community – shared energy and structures to guide its practice. Notably, distinctive spiritual care traditions (e.g., Buddhist and Jewish spiritual care) hold many commonalities with one another – including the shared calling to uphold spiritual health, even if they define such health in variable ways. Various spiritual care traditions hence can and should draw from and mutually support one another. This is currently practiced in many spiritual care departments in health care institutions where chaplains from many different spiritual traditions (including 'spiritual not religious' and other non-traditional perspectives) can mutually support and encourage one another in a common vocation of spiritual care practice. However, even still, disparate spiritual traditions have distinct communal sources

(Tracy Balboni 2013). Hence, each spiritual care tradition must be sourced in its unique spiritual community, as only herein lies the requisite communal life, energy, vision, and structure that can robustly enliven that tradition's spiritual care practice.

Having set the foundation of the source for spiritual care – a community embodying a shared vision and structure for spiritual life – we turn to considering the particular source of Christian spiritual care. Returning to Jesus' words – "your faith has made you well" – faith is here named as the source of healing. But what is meant by 'faith'? Christian faith is one's self-commitment and self-surrender to the triune God – the community of the Father, Son and Holy Spirit. And with that faith comes entry into the life of that community, and in so doing entry into the community of all Christian believers – the body of Christ (1 Corinthians 12:27). Hence, in Jesus' words we see that the source of all spiritual healing (and the resultant practice of spiritual care) emanates from the Community of God accessed and indwelled by one's faith. Christian spiritual care – all its life, energy, and structures – must be sourced in the divine community of the Father, Son and Holy Spirit accessed and experienced through the mystery of faith.

Therefore, Christian spiritual care – the nurturing of Christian spiritual health – must be centered on faith as the passageway to the divine community where spiritual life was borne and is sustained. This spiritual care foundation of faith begins with the spiritual caregiver themselves. Spiritual caregivers must be continually nurtured in their faith and communal life with the Triune God. This means they themselves ground their spiritual caregiving in the support of personal prayer and meditation on scripture – manifesting a continual individual surrender of one's life and vocation to God and his Word. Jesus, the Great Physician and the Great Spiritual Caregiver, himself withdrew for the regular practice of prayer (Luke 5:16). Moreover, his intimate knowledge of scripture is reflected in his words (not to mention, he himself is the Word, John 1:14). Furthermore, the spiritual caregiver must have a life faithfully committed to a community of Christian faith, sharing in sacred practices (e.g., communion) as well as sharing life together, including the burdens and joys of spiritual caregiving with fellow believers. Christian spiritual care practice should be additionally buttressed by dedicated time for personal receipt of spiritual care where there can be reflection on one's own faith, particularly as it intersects with the practice of spiritual caregiving. Just as psychiatrists and psychologists typically have a regular practice of personal counselling for sharing their own journeys and trials as mental health practitioners, Christian spiritual caregivers should have a dedicated person or group with whom to share the trials and joys of spiritual caregiving together with personal reflection on one's own faith journey.

Christian spiritual care of the ill person should likewise be grounded in this source – the community of the triune God – experienced through faith. The center of Christian spiritual care should hence be the exploration and illumination of the nature of the person's Christian faith, including identifying places of strength, fragmentation and potential transformation. Furthermore, faith practices of personal prayer, scriptural meditation, and communal life and sacraments, are to be a framework for Christian spiritual care, as the primary structures to an individual and collective faith. Like the frame and hinges of a door, so are prayer, scripture and communal life and practices to the door that is faith – faith cannot function without their supportive framing.

The spiritual caregiver is called upon first and foremost to assist the ill person to be challenged to a new, renewed, and/or deepening faith – the very source of connection to the dynamic life of God and the body of Christ. Without this source, all efforts toward Christian spiritual health are futile. Dwelling within this source – faith that enters us into the communal life of the triune God – we are made whole, "your faith has made you well."

4 The Mode of Christian Spiritual Care

Having considered the source of Christian spiritual care – the divine communal life of the triune God experienced through faith – we next consider the mode of Christian spiritual care and healing. By mode, we consider the method or mechanism by which healing occurs. To again provide a conceptual analogy, we turn to consider the physical mode of healing as an illustration. In physical healing, the mode is through the recognition and targeting of sources of injury and the restoration of these processes to their original wholeness. As an example, the healing of cancer requires the identification of the bodily tissues that have developed distorted and nefarious growth patterns, such as unchecked growth to the detriment of surrounding normal tissues and dissemination to other sites of the body. Surgery, systemic therapies, and/or radiation therapy are then utilized to target those cells – tools that preferentially destroy aberrant cells. After a process of normal tissue healing after the injury sustained by cancer treatment – if cure has been achieved – the body's cellular tissues resume their original pattern of appropriately checked growth that results in the restoration of health of the entire person. Wholeness has been restored.

Having considered the physical mode of healing, we turn to the spiritual mode of healing. As God is the source of physical healing, like a mirror, the patterns of spiritual healing are closely related (Tracy Balboni and Balboni 2018).

Like the physical, spiritual healing similarly involves the restoration of the originally intended processes of spiritual life, requiring the identification and undoing of spiritual processes that are distorted, fragmented or destroyed. It is perhaps for this reason that Jesus says, "your faith has *made* you well." The verb for "made well" or "made whole" is the Greek *sozo*, which can either refer to a rescue of physical deliverance or in terms of transcendent salvation (Arndt et al. 2000). As the gospel records Jesus' words, it seems clear that his intention in the physical act of healing simultaneously signals a spiritual salvation. Faith yields healing in body, relationship, and soul.

In reflecting biblically on *sozo*, we readily see that the mode of spiritual healing simultaneously hearkens back to the original wholeness found in the Genesis creation story while also pointing toward the wholeness found in the future new creation as illustrated in Revelation. To picture 'original spiritual health' we look back to creation and our pre-fall state – Adam and Eve dwelling in communion with God in the Garden of Eden. There we see right relationship to God, to one another, and to the surrounding environment. Physical, emotional, social, intellectual and spiritual health are wholly integrated and functioning in mutually beneficial concert.

Yet sin enters this picture as a distortion of the heart's properly ordered desires created by God. These desires, though good, result in spiritual disease and death when they supersede the primary importance of love of God. Included in Genesis 3 are distortions of right desires for: (1) physical good ('the tree was . . . good for food', Gen 3:6), (2) emotional good in the form of beauty ('the tree was . . . a delight to the eyes', Gen 3:6), (3) intellectual good in the form of wisdom ('the tree was . . . to be desired to make one wise', Gen 3:6), and (4) social good in the form of desiring social harmony and communion ('. . . she also gave some to her husband who was with her, and he ate', Gen 3:6). And preeminently, we see the distorted desire for spiritual good ('you will be like God', Gen 3:5). The heart's improperly ordered desires break close relationship with God (Gen 3:8). All together these yield physical, relational, and spiritual death.

And yet, looking forward, there is hope for restoration and renewal of spiritual life. Revelation 21:4 promises, "He will wipe away every tear from their eyes, and death shall be no more, neither shall there be mourning, nor crying, nor pain anymore, for the former things have passed away. And he who was seated on the throne said, 'Behold, I am making all things new.'" Physical healing brought about by the energies of the medical community, whether the healing of a skin rash or the resuscitation of a person in cardiac arrest, reflects the ultimate physical healing that will come through death and resurrection in Christ. Similarly, spiritual healing in the context of Christian spiritual care, however incremental or transformative, foreshadows the ultimate spiritual health and renewal that will come through Christ's sacrifice, resurrection and return.

The mode of spiritual healing, therefore, involves recognition of sources of spiritual fragmentation from the originally created wholeness – including physical, emotional, intellectual, social, and/or spiritual distortions – whether those personally committed and/or those unjustly suffered. But though spiritual fragmentation must be recognized and addressed, we do not remain there. Rather, in Christian spiritual care the center and heart is the truth that we are children of God, and no matter how marred by sin and injustice, there is the undeniable hope of the spiritual restoration to come. Hence, healing within Christian spiritual care comes through the recognition of the dignity and beauty of the person because they are made in God's glorious image. Furthermore, healing comes through the embrace of the new creation each person is in Christ, now a seed, but one day will effloresce into the whole and glorious creation the person is destined to become in resurrection life (1 Corinthians 15:42–49).

In summary, the mode of Christian healing involves (1) the recognition and addressing of spiritual fragmentation from our original, God-reflecting wholeness, and (2) the upholding of the person as a new creation in Christ. What does this mode of healing within Christian spiritual care practically look like? Christian spiritual care communities are called upon to ponder this, and depending on the cultural context and theological emphases, modes of Christian spiritual healing will manifest in variable ways. That said, thoughtful scholarship in spiritual care provides some essential practical pieces of that framework. For example, we know that spiritual fragmentation, termed spiritual needs in the research literature, are common in the setting of illness and variable in type (Riklikienė et al. 2019; Astrow et al. 2018). Christian spiritual care should involve the assessment of spiritual needs, whether utilizing survey tools or other frameworks (Büssing, Balzat, and Heusser 2010), and the addressing of those needs.

5 The Goal of Christian Spiritual Care

Having considered the source and mode of Christian spiritual care, we now turn to its goal. Previously, we have named the goal as wholeness. In the prior section, this was illustrated with the physical care example of the cure of a malignancy. However, continuing in the vein of this example, if we step back and take a wider view of the state of the person cured of cancer, we see a larger and more primary issue. The person is, despite this cure, destined for death. Our efforts to bring healing here on earth – though very good and worthy of our deep commitment –

are never sufficient, they never 'cure' the more primary issue – the sure fate of death.

This primary issue of the deeper need for healing must be at the center of Christian spiritual care. When Jesus says, "Your faith has made you well," he does not simply mean that faith has been the source of the specific physical healing received, whether sight restored, hemorrhage stopped, or leprosy healed. Rather, Jesus repeats this statement in the context of healing to counter the tendency to believe that bodily healing is all that is in view. Jesus is calling us to see the physical manifestation of healing as a pointer to the preeminent goal of finding complete wholeness in the triune God through faith. Though only a small proportion of the many persons with physical ailments who came to Jesus were healed, in proclaiming, "your faith has made you well," Jesus reveals that this ultimate healing is available to all. Wholeness remains available in faith to the woman with the bloody discharge, the healed blind man, and the man healed of leprosy who all subsequently physically suffered and died, perhaps not long after their temporary healings. Wholeness remains available to all who in faith rest in the community of the triune God who is the source of all life.

Hence, following the pattern set and proclaimed by Jesus, Christian spiritual care must have as its primary goal wholeness in the triune God. This includes a right and good hope for physical healing not as the end goal but rather as a pointer to this ultimate goal. This may manifest itself as personal prayers for physical healing (even in the face of unbelief, Mark 9:23–24), corporate prayers for healing and anointing by elders (James 5:14), and/or as physical healing by way of repentance of sin (Mark 2:9–12; John 5:14). But physical healing is a sign and symbol of the need for wholeness in the triune God. What then does wholeness in God look like? What is the goal to which we, including all Christian spiritual care, should hope? Jesus "the author and perfecter of our faith" (Hebrews 12:2) is our goal. Jesus is the one who continually dwelled in the source as he communed with the Father. Jesus is the one whose life on earth was characterized by continual emblems of the restoration of all things:

> And the scroll of the prophet Isaiah was given to him. He unrolled the scroll and found the place where it was written,
>
> 'The Spirit of the Lord is upon me, because he has anointed me to proclaim good news to the poor. He has sent me to proclaim liberty to the captives and recovering of sight to the blind, to set at liberty those who are oppressed, to proclaim the year of the Lord's favor.'
>
> And he rolled up the scroll and gave it back to the attendant and sat down. And the eyes of all in the synagogue were fixed on him. And he began saying to them. 'Today this Scripture has been fulfilled in your hearing.' Luke 4:17–21

And finally, despite suffering physical, emotional, intellectual, social and ultimately spiritual suffering and death, Christ rose again as firstborn of the new creation. He has himself brought about the final healing; he is the new creation – the ultimate wholeness in which lies our hope. Hence, the goal of Christian spiritual care is Christ himself – the one and only who has dwelled in the source, restores all broken things, and has brought in himself through the cross – the darkest depths of sin – wholeness in God. Jesus beckons us to hope in this ultimate reality that despite the darkness of this earthly life, "your faith has made you whole."

6 Christian Spiritual Care and Healing of Health Care

Having examined the source, mode, and goal of Christian spiritual care, we now turn to consider the practical implications of these greater realities on daily clinical practice. Furthermore, we will consider how the practice of Christian spiritual care holds promise to bring healing and restoration to the larger practice of health care. To do these things, we return to the case of Carol, concluding the story of her and her husband John's care:

In response to John's statement about his belief in a miracle for Carol, Daniel, the radiation oncologist, says to him, "I see that you and Ms. James have a spirituality that's important to you. Would you tell me more about that?" John proceeds to explain that he and his wife were nominal Catholics prior to her diagnosis, but her cancer prompted a spiritual "revival" for them. He describes how they have never been closer in their marriage as they've gotten closer to God together through her illness. He also notes that they believe in medical science, but ultimately, it is, "God who has removed the cancer from her body." He then again reiterates how he believes God can do this again because he believes in "a God of miracles."

The physician, Daniel, finished residency training two years ago and took a faculty job at the hospital – a large academic hospital on the East Coast – where he did his training. He grew up in Alabama, attending a Baptist church with his family, but didn't become a Christian until the beginning of medical school after he was admitted for severe depression and suicidality – a crisis that caused him to reexamine the Christian faith and led to a conversion experience. He regularly attends a vibrant Bethel AME church in the city where he works. Several fellow congregants work at the same hospital, including nurses, doctors, medical assistants and environmental services staff. He received spiritual care training in his medical school that included shadowing a chaplain for several days which he deeply enjoyed. In residency training, Daniel did not receive ongoing training in how to provide spiritual care to cancer patients, so he elected to attend a 1-day seminar on providing Christian spiritual care in health care about six months prior to meeting John and Carol. This helped Daniel to deepen his spiritual care skills and the integration of his faith with his work, something he has been sharing with his small group Bible study.

Using these spiritual care skills, Daniel responds to John's sharing of his and his wife's faith and their belief in miracles by saying, "Thank you for sharing about your and your wife's faith. It's clear it has brought you both a lot of comfort as you've dealt with her cancer. I also so appreciate your sharing your belief in miracles; I also hope for a miracle for Mrs. James. As your radiation oncologist, I want to make sure I provide you with all the information you need to make a decision about her treatment. Can you help me to begin in the right place by telling me your and your wife's understanding of her illness?"

John pauses for a moment and then shares that his wife Carol, "knows she is going to die. "He pauses again and says, "She said to me before they put the tube in that she's ready to go . . . that I need to let her go. I just can't." He begins to cry. Daniel puts his hand on his shoulder and says, "I'm sorry this is so hard. I can tell you love your wife very much." John responds, "I don't want to see her suffer like this. I just can't imagine living without her. I thought God would have me die first. Not her. Why does this have to happen to her?" There is a long silence, and then Daniel asks, "I know your faith is very important to you and to Mrs. James. Would it be ok if I asked the Catholic chaplain to come?" John nods, and says, "Yes, I think both of us need that."

The Catholic chaplain is called and happens to be nearby in the ICU finishing a meeting with a patient and family. Catherine is a woman in her late 40s, with a doctorate in the health sciences. She considered religious life for several years, even spending one year as a novitiate in a convent. She discerned at the end of that year a calling to remain in health care and become a chaplain. After finishing the appropriate training, she began working as a chaplain four years ago at this hospital. She also acts as a preceptor for the medical student course that includes training in spiritual care, and medical students frequently are shadowing her in the hospital. Her spiritual practices include attending mass multiple times per week, she is actively serving in her Catholic parish, and she has a spiritual director with whom she has been sharing her spiritual life, challenges, and growths, including in her work as a chaplain. Catherine steps in and Daniel excuses himself, saying he'll return later.

Catherine speaks to John about his and his wife Carol's faith journey. She hears from John about Carol's strong faith and how she had calmly said to him, just an hour before she was intubated, that she is at peace with dying and that she knows, "where I'm going." John then indicates he knows too where she is going, but he, "just can't imagine letting her go." "I can't imagine life without her," he says with tears in his eyes. Catherine also explores with John what he's heard from Carol's medical caregivers and suggests that they have a family meeting to discuss what might be the best next steps in her medical care. John agrees.

Over the next two days, Catherine brings practices of prayer to Carol and prayer and communion to John, who remains in the ICU family waiting area or at Carol's bedside. Carol's nurses provide respectful space for prayer at the bedside. Jenny, Carol's ICU nurse who has been on the day shift since Carol arrived, is Presbyterian by background but has since a teenager no longer been attending services. She considers herself 'spiritual not religious' though attends services at her parents' Presbyterian church a few times a year for holidays, such as Easter. Jenny finds these times of Catherine's prayers at the bedside deeply meaningful, particularly in the midst of the hard and tragic realities she sees in the ICU. Just two days prior to Carol's arrival, she cared for a young man, Tom, with leukemia in his mid-30s – the same age as Jenny. He died unexpectantly due to complications of his curative treatment despite the ICU team's valiant efforts to save him. After Tom's death and after a few other recent difficult patient cases, Jenny has had meaningful conversations with Catherine, who is a frequent presence in the ICU. Catherine invited Jenny to take part in the staff spiritual care events she and other chaplains lead for the ICU staff, and Jenny has now attended a few of these. Catherine recently led one of these events the day after Tom died. Jenny was surprised when she found herself crying during this time. She had cried on occasion after tough patient cases early in her career as an ICU nurse, but now 8 years into her career, she felt hardened, even numb, to the tragedies she saw. Covid-19 – and the many dying patients she cared for and watched die without loved ones – only had deepened that numbness, and she had strongly been considering quitting nursing. The fact that she and her partner needed her salary to cover their mortgage was all that had been keeping her in her position as an ICU nurse.

Carol's three children arrive and take turns with their father spending time at their mother's bedside. Their parish priest, Father Steven, also visits the family. Carol's physical condition gradually worsens – she is requiring more medications to support her blood pressure, and her kidneys are showing signs of failure. A family meeting is held with John and his three children, and includes Catherine the chaplain, the primary oncologist, Daniel the radiation oncologist, and the ICU attending, resident, and Jenny the nurse. The medical team speaks to Carol's prognosis, which is very poor, rendering all cancer interventions unlikely to extend her life and more likely to prolong her suffering. There is a long silence after this information is shared, and the family is asked if they have any questions. Catherine then speaks to what John shared about his wife – Carol's strong faith in God, her peace and readiness as demonstrated in her words to John prior to her intubation. This sharing brings hopefulness and even joy into the family meeting, which otherwise thus far had seemed devoid of hope. John and his three children speak of Carol lovingly and share tearfully how they each know that she is ready, and they must "let go" of her. The ICU team explains the next steps in their medical care supporting Carol's symptoms to keep her comfortable. Catherine speaks to John and his children about how she will support them through this time, including notifying Father Steven to perform Carol's last rites. Carol dies peacefully that evening with John and her three children and Father Steven at her bedside.

This story – taken from pieces of true events of multiple patient and family stories – illustrates the source, mode, and goal of Christian spiritual care in many dimensions. First, we see Catherine's spiritual care for John and Carol. Ironically, though Carol is the 'sick person' of the story, she is the most spiritually healthy. In fact, from the greater Christian spiritual care perspective, she is arguably the most alive. She has come to a place of peace and feels ready and hopeful in death. Rather, it is John who is spiritually struggling and needs healing. Hence, Catherine focuses Christian spiritual care for him, calling him to deeper faith in God through prayer and communion, even as she provides ongoing spiritual care for Carol as she journeys through her final days to death. Spiritual care is also given to the entire family, in Catherine's presence with the three children and in her presence and words at the family meeting. These words brought Carol's Christian spiritual life into the meeting in a way that engenders hopefulness and greater freedom for the family in "letting go". Catherine's Christian spiritual care is also seen in her role in connecting the family to the Jones' parish priest, Father Steven, during the hospital stay. Fostering connections with spiritual supporters in the community is central to ensuring community grounded spiritual care, and to fostering ongoing spiritual care after patients and families leave the medical setting.

In addition to caring for patients and families, Catherine is also seen providing spiritual care for the medical staff, including through her presence to them and to the patients and families in the ICU. This is particularly seen in Jenny, an ICU nurse who has been experiencing emotional exhaustion and spiritual struggle in the setting of witnessing suffering and tragedy, including Tom's recent death. We also see the indirect way that Catherine's Christian spiritual care allows Daniel, the radiation oncologist, to play his own role as a generalist Christian spiritual caregiver (Puchalski et al. 2014). Catherine, together with other chaplains of many traditions, participates as a preceptor for a spiritual care course that allows medical students like Daniel to witness and practice spiritual care skills. Furthermore, we see Daniel taking the initiative to deepen his Christian spiritual care skills and to ground his vocation in personal and communal faith practices. With Daniel playing his role as a Christian spiritual care generalist and recognizing the need for specialist spiritual care early in Carol's admission, Catherine is able to more fully play her role as a Christian spiritual caregiver to Carol, John, their children, and to the medical team.

Catherine's Christian spiritual care is grounded in her own regular spiritual practices of worship in mass, participation in her religious community, and dedicated time with her spiritual director with whom she shares her faith journey and struggles, including those she faces in her chaplaincy work. Moreover, Catherine's spiritual care is a living manifestation of Jesus's proclamation that, "your faith has made you well." It is sourced in faith in the triune God. It is centered on helping patients and families like Carol and John, as well as staff like Jenny, to grow in faith and to lay places of brokenness before God through personal and communal spiritual practices. It also points patients and families like Carol, John and their children and the entire medical team to a hopefulness that transcends death, as beautifully illustrated by Catherine's testimony of Carol's flourishing Christian spiritual life as she approaches death.

Finally, Christian spiritual care, and spiritual care's integration into medical care more generally, has an important role in supporting and healing healthcare systems (Tracy Anne Balboni et al. 2022). This is evident in this case as it illustrates how spiritual care can provide needed support to clinicians, particularly for those facing burnout (Whitehead et al. 2023). Furthermore, in this case, it is evident how spiritual care can impact medical decision-making and care for patients and their families. For example, Daniel's spiritual history-taking and referral to chaplaincy led to Catherine addressing urgent spiritual care needs, influencing the surrogate decision-maker John. One can imagine what could have happened had Daniel simply proceeded with radiation therapy for Carol without addressing the issues underlying John's hope for a miracle for Carol. In studies of terminally ill patients and their families, religious beliefs in end-of-life care are common, and can influence medical care decisions (Tracy Anne Balboni et al. 2019; Bülow et al. 2012; Silvestri et al. 2003).

Furthermore, when spiritual care is provided to patients and families, patients tend to receive greater comfort-focused end-of-life medical care, patients have better quality of life near death, and families have better well-being and care satisfaction (Torke et al. 2023; Tracy Anne Balboni et al. 2010). Spiritual care hence has a critical role to play in supporting health care systems, and in particular for Christian spiritual care, in providing a vibrant witness to the mysterious, ultimate reality that it is faith that makes us whole.

7 Conclusion

In summary, Christ's proclamation, "your faith has made you well" shapes a practice of Christian spiritual care sourced in faith in the triune God, centered on personal and communal practices of restoration of brokenness and pointing to the hope of wholeness that is found in Christ, the firstborn of the new creation. In so doing, Christian patients and families are drawn into the vibrant life of the community of the triune God, a source that brings restoration of brokenness and hope in the new life through Christ who has conquered death. Moreover, as salt to the world, Christian spiritual care brings to the health care community a source of healing of its own wounds from bearing the burdens of caring for those who suffer physical illness and a source of hope far greater than the limited hopes of physical healing. Together with Jesus, Christian spiritual care proclaims to patients, their families and communities, and health systems, "your faith has made you well."

References

Arndt, W, FW Danker, W Bauer, and FW Gingrich. 2000. 'Sozo'. In A Greek-English Lexicon of the New Testament and Other Early Christian Literature, 3rd ed., 982. Chicago, IL: University of Chicago Press.

Astrow, Alan B, Gary Kwok, Rashmi K Sharma, Nelli Fromer, and Daniel P. Sulmasy. 2018. 'Spiritual Needs and Perception of Quality of Care and Satisfaction with Care in Hematology/Medical Oncology Patients: A Multicultural Assessment'. Journal of Pain and Symptom Management 55 (1): 56-64.e1. https://doi.org/10.1016/j.jpainsymman.2017.08.009.

Balboni, Michael J. 2013. 'A Theological Assessment of Spiritual Assessments'. Christian Bioethics: Non-Ecumenical Studies in Medical Morality 19 (3): 313–31. https://doi.org/10.1093/cb/cbt023.

Balboni, Michael J, and Tracy A Balboni. 2018. Hostility to Hospitality: Spirituality and Professional Socialization within Medicine. Oxford, UK: Oxford University Press.

Balboni, Tracy A, Holly G. Prigerson, Michael J Balboni, Andrea C Enzinger, Tyler J VanderWeele, and Paul K Maciejewski. 2019. 'A Scale to Assess Religious Beliefs in End-of-Life Medical Care'. Cancer 125 (9): 1527–35. https://doi.org/10.1002/cncr.31946.

Balboni, Tracy A, Tyler J Van der Weele, Stephanie D Doan-Soares, Katelyn NG Long, Betty R Ferrell, George Fitchett, Harold G Koenig, Paul A Bain, Christina Puchalski, and Karen E Steinhauser. 2022. 'Spirituality in Serious Illness and Health'. Journal of the American Medical Association 328 (2): 184–97.

Balboni, Tracy Anne, Mary Elizabeth Paulk, Michael J Balboni, Andrea C Phelps, Elizabeth Trice Loggers, Alexi A Wright, Susan D Block, Eldrin F Lewis, John R Peteet, and Holly Gwen Prigerson. 2010. 'Provision of Spiritual Care to Patients with Advanced Cancer: Associations with Medical Care and Quality of Life near Death'. Journal of Clinical Oncology 28 (3): 445–52.

Bülow, Hans-Henrik, Charles L Sprung, Mario Baras, Sara Carmel, Mia Svantesson, Julie Benbenishty, Paulo A Maia, Albertus Beishuizen, Simon Cohen, and Daniel Nalos. 2012. 'Are Religion and

Religiosity Important to End-of-Life Decisions and Patient Autonomy in the ICU? The Ethicatt Study'. Intensive Care Medicine 38:1126–33.

Büssing, A, HJ Balzat, and P Heusser. 2010. 'Spiritual Needs of Patients with Chronic Pain Diseases and Cancer – Validation of the Spiritual Needs Questionnaire'. European Journal of Medical Research 15 (6): 266–73. https://doi.org/10.1186/2047-783x-15-6-266.

Puchalski, Christina M, Robert Vitillo, Sharon K Hull, and Nancy Reller. 2014. 'Improving the Spiritual Dimension of Whole Person Care: Reaching National and International Consensus'. Journal of Palliative Medicine 17 (6): 642–56. https://doi.org/10.1089/jpm.2014.9427.

Riklikienė, Olga,Jūratė Tomkevičiūtė, Lina Spirgienė, Žaneta Valiulienė, and Arndt Büssing. 2019. 'Spiritual Needs and Their Association with Indicators of Quality of Life among Non-Terminally Ill Cancer Patients: Cross-Sectional Survey'. European Journal of Oncology Nursing 44. https://www.ejoncologynursing.com/article/S1462-3889(19)30149-8/fulltext.

Silvestri, Gerard A, Sommer Knittig, James S Zoller, and Paul J Nietert. 2003. 'Importance of Faith on Medical Decisions Regarding Cancer Care'. Journal of Clinical Oncology 21 (7): 1379–82.

Torke, Alexia M, Shelley E Varner-Perez, Emily S Burke, Tracy A Taylor, James E Slaven, Kathryn L Kozinski, Saneta M Maiko, Bruce J Pfeffer, and Sarah K Banks. 2023. 'Effects of Spiritual Care on Well-Being of Intensive Care Family Surrogates: A Clinical Trial'. Journal of Pain and Symptom Management 65 (4): 296–307.

Whitehead, Ishbel Orla, Suzanne Moffatt, Stephanie Warwick, Gemma F. Spiers, Tafadzwa Patience Kunonga, Eugene Tang, and Barbara Hanratty. 2023. 'Systematic Review of the Relationship between Burn-out and Spiritual Health in Doctors'. BMJ Open 13 (8): e068402. https://doi.org/10.1136/bmjopen-2022-068402.

Annette Haußmann

Why Research Matters. Preservation and Transformation of Christian Healthcare Chaplaincy in Germany

Abstract: This contribution reflects on the current transformation processes within hospital chaplaincy in Germany, drawing insights from case vignettes of pastoral care practice. It highlights tensions between hospital chaplaincy as specialized pastoral care and parish related pastoral care, emphasizing the need to conceptualize the health-promoting dimension of pastoral care more broadly as part of congregational work and a community-oriented church. Particular potentials lie in outpatient care, especially given the reduced hospital stays and the increasing need for measures of health prevention. An interprofessionally connected hospital chaplaincy can provide valuable input in this context. This chapter argues that there is a need to foster empirical research on hospital chaplaincy, to enhance knowledge about its effectiveness and role in healthcare. In an environment primarily driven by empirical evidence and efficacy in hospital economics, hospital chaplaincy must position itself transparently and confidently, with high-quality empirical research playing a crucial role. Emphasizing the importance of a detailed focus on lived spirituality is particularly crucial, including the perspective of healthcare chaplains in shaping their personal and professional identity. Looking ahead, this chapter addresses the future challenges and opportunities, discussing the concept of outreaching chaplaincy and the prospective financing of healthcare chaplaincy.

1 Healthcare Chaplaincy From an Interdisciplinary and Interprofessional Perspective

I am not a hospital chaplain myself, but I am rooted in two disciplines and two professions. I studied Protestant theology and psychology and later specialized in Practical Theology with my dissertation on the transformation and ambivalence of lived religion in the context of family caregiving (Haussmann 2019). On a professional level, I am also trained as a psychotherapist, with a focus on Cognitive Behavioural Therapy (CBT). During my training, for approximately five years I worked with patients, their relatives and other professionals in the healthcare system, including outpatient therapy in my training institutes in Tübingen and Munich, and in a clinic for psychiatry and psychotherapy at the Ludwig-

https://doi.org/10.1515/9783112205839-005

Maximilian-University in Munich. In the psychiatric clinic, I offered therapy to patients on a regular basis at least once, mostly twice a week, according to their individual needs and the severity of symptoms. Additionally, I have also led group therapies. Our ward was not specialized in a certain psychiatric disorder. Thus, we had a broad range of patients of all ages and different types of mental illnesses, which made my work very interesting and challenging at the same time.

Today, I have paused my therapeutic work to concentrate on my professorship in practical theology and pastoral care at Heidelberg University, where I work since 2019 , first as a junior professor and then tenured since 2025. My research is focused on the empirical research on religion and spirituality and also explores practices of pastoral care in a pluralistic society, in digital communication, and in respect to interprofessional collaboration. I am interested in the dialogue between CBT and pastoral/spiritual care, and the question of what theology and psychology can learn from each other in general. Part of my teaching activities is the training in pastoral care for future pastors of the regional Protestant Church in Baden, which is located in the south of Germany. As the director of the Centre for Pastoral Care (Zentrum für Seelsorge), I am also responsible for developing new trainings for professionals and volunteers specializing in various areas of pastoral care, ranging from congregational work to hospital chaplaincy.

Concerning healthcare chaplaincy and its current developments, I will be discussing and reflecting from an external perspective (as a psychotherapist) and from an internal perspective (as a theologian and researcher). I will answer these questions with my threefold background in scientific research (1) within the domains of practical theology, psychology of religion/spirituality and psychotherapy; (2) with regard to my professional perspective on the healthcare system as a psychotherapist, and (3) considering my work in pastoral care training and research, and development of these trainings.

2 Tensions and Conflicts Between Hospital Chaplaincy and Church Congregations

2.1 Two Vignettes from German Healthcare Chaplaincy

A) *“We need more pastoral care in palliative care”*

In summer 2022, I gave a seminar on pastoral care and palliative/spiritual care at Heidelberg University. Students were asked to visit the palliative care ward in the local clinic in Heidelberg, with only 10 beds for terminally ill patients. The healthcare chaplain was also part of the seminar and participated in some of the seminar meetings. He was a part-time hospital chaplain with 25% of his work-time and spent the rest of the week as a pastor in the local church congregation. His colleague, a female social worker, accompanied him to one seminar meeting and explained her view on hospital chaplaincy. She was really convinced of its importance, not only to the patients and their relatives, but also for the team. Two years ago, she would explain, they had a 50% hospital chaplain that worked part-time in the hospital and part-time in the local church congregation. He would be present a in the hospital, talking to patients and staff, sharing their joys and sorrows. Now that only 25% of the chaplaincy position remained, there was little time for staff meetings and concerns. Two days each week, he visited some of the patients and participates in team meetings. The chaplain himself regretted the situation and would have loved to be present more often, but his duties in the church congregation were equally important to him. The social worker concluded: "now that it is only 25% health care chaplaincy, only a fraction of the conversations with patients are possible compared to before. There are also fewer joint meetings and rituals such as blessings, and end-of-life care. All these tasks cannot simply be taken over by the other professions, they disappear or have to be compensated for in some other way. But we need a strong hospital chaplaincy!"

B) *Team-integrated hospital chaplaincy supported by the clinic*

Another healthcare chaplain works full-time in the general hospital and is available for patients and staff all of her working time. However, she is intensively involved in the processes and structures of the hospital management. She is present in the daily rounds in the ward and in the team meetings. They discuss disease progressions, and the chaplain is closely involved in current developments. This is only possible because the clinic's senior physician highly appreciates pastoral care and encourages all healthcare chaplains to engage in extended activities in the clinic. Therefore, the chaplain is also part of the clinic's ethics committee – as was her predecessor, who was involved in many ethical decisions, especially during the Covid-19 pandemic. In addition, she is present on the wards assigned to her through outreach pastoral care by going to the patients' rooms and actively offering the patients her time, being there and listening. When asked about her understanding of her role as a hospital chaplain, she acknowledged that, of course, she finds it challenging to leave her office and actively approach patients to offer pastoral care. Because she never knows what awaits her behind a door, and whether her offer will be appreciated or rejected. She also pointed out a certain conflict between "outreaching" pastoral care and the hospital's organizational structure: since she is well known and appreciated at her hospital, it would be possible to spend the whole day in team meetings, resulting in less time to actively visit patients in their rooms. However, she views this outreaching, visiting aspect of her work as essential and vital, and she does not wish to exclude it from her chaplaincy practice.

2.2 Specialization and Professionalization in Health Care Chaplaincy

To understand the differences between both vignettes described above, the specific nature of hospital chaplaincy in Germany and its historical developments have to be taken into account. The history of hospital chaplaincy in Germany is characterized by ongoing professionalization and specialization (Klessmann 2019) – like most other professions nowadays.

On the one hand, this specialization is important and necessary because the healthcare system is becoming increasingly complex. On the other hand, the hospital pastorate is increasingly characterized by generalization, i.e., more and more different tasks are added to the job description so that it increasingly resembles the parish pastorate in its structure (Peng-Keller 2021). This also bespeaks the necessity for chaplains to constantly evaluate where their work and presence is most needed and does the greatest good. Two characteristics of the hospital chaplaincy in Germany make it difficult and at the same time easier to bring the duality of the two roles into dialogue with each other.

Firstly, it is common for pastors to take up work in the hospital sector only after a long period of training in the vicariate and probationary service, as well as a certain time in the parish pastorate. This means that pastors who work in clinics have usually formed a strong identity in the parish ministry and only then find their way into the healthcare system. The path is, of course, accompanied by training in pastoral care (usually: clinical pastoral care training, KSA/CPE), which is costly and time-consuming. Many clinical pastor positions are also limited to part-time, so they run parallel to the parish pastorate. In these cases, it is up to the pastors themselves how they organize their work in the congregation and in the clinic – and they are not necessarily well-trained in pastoral care. As a rule, they are present in the clinic for one or two days to offer pastoral care, rituals, and the like.

In my seminars taught at Heidelberg University, I experience the students as highly interested in pastoral and spiritual care. This is also reflected in the few studies on the motivations of theology students: their faith and the desire to offer pastoral care and support to others often are their primary motivation for studying theology (Baden 2020). I am often asked whether it is possible to specialize in pastoral care or clinical pastoral care at an early stage in theological education. Some students are already involved in pastoral care on a voluntary basis, most commonly in youth work, as emergency chaplains or voluntary hospital chaplains. This potential resource is wasted if specialization is only possible at a late stage of professional development. At the same time, early specialization would be appropriate in the increasingly complex system of hospitals and healthcare. The age structure of the chaplains could also change in a positive way (I am thinking for example of the positive reactions on the palliative ward of the elderly patients towards young pastoral care students). Secondly, the church – I am referring here to the Protestant Church in Germany, which is losing more and more members and attracts ever fewer young people to study theology – can no longer afford expanding into the specialized areas of pastoral care because it is struggling to maintain full coverage with chaplains for church congregations. Especially in the north-eastern regions of Germany, there are some areas with one pastor serving up to 20 church parishes. Due to demographic changes, a decreasing number of church members, retiring pastoral staff and fewer students of theology, the church needs to adapt.

The conflict concerning hospital chaplaincy is that church leaders seem to focus mainly on the religious life in church congregations, which also sometimes seems to lead to a certain reluctance to provide pastoral care training for their pastors. In the Protestant Church in Baden (a regional church in the south of Germany), a total of 30% of all parish posts will be cut by 2030. It was decided to treat all areas of church life equally, regardless of their relevance, thus also affecting hospital chaplaincy in a central manner. The few hospital chaplains already have so much to do in the hospitals that a further reduction in employment positions can only lead to poorer pastoral care for patients.

2.3 Towards a Model of Integrating Healthcare and Congregational Work

A characteristic of pastoral care is that it can approach people and actively offer its services to them or simply meet people in very different life situations. This is true in church congregations, but also in schools, in nursing homes or even in hospital chaplaincy. Such encounters can either be actively initiated or occur spontaneously because they are about life as such and therefore also concern healthcare issues. This is an enormous opportunity to maintain a pastoral care service independent of the setting, to offer spiritual and psychosocial support both in the clinic and then to continue it in congregational contexts. Pastoral care can therefore be seen as highly relevant for healthcare in different fields of pastoral work, from church congregation to hospitals.

This has advantages for the role of hospital chaplains between the church and the health care system: Through the non-permanent commitment to the healthcare system or the simultaneity of congregational work and hospital chaplaincy (see vignette A), there is the possibility of networking with the congregational work and regional healthcare providers (e.g., general practitioners or counselling services) Leerzeile ergänzen. The identity of chaplains therefore becomes twofold: they are members of the healthcare system, but also represent a specific faith community by having a role as pastor and member of the congregation. This could strengthen their self-identification of belonging to both systems – but can also challenge them. Chaplains could serve as 'boundary workers'– linking the community and the institution of care.

On the other hand, there are also fundamental disadvantages: our study on pastoral care during the Covid-19 pandemic in Germany suggested that in order to maintain pastoral care in hospitals, above all, the permanent presence of hospital chaplains is central to their successful work (see vignette B). Chaplains who only held part-time positions of 25% or 50% were much more quickly excluded from the healthcare system: they were no longer provided access or were simply not included in the internal discussions and processes. This happened because they were not always known to the hospital staff, but also simply because their work of pastoral care was not perceived as relevant. However, when hospital chaplains were intensively involved in the healthcare teams, not only was seamless pastoral work possible, but the chaplains were also intensively involved in internal processes, such as ethical decision-making or care for Covid-19 patients. This clearly shows how important it is for the chaplains to be integrated in the hospital system in order to be able to work continuously and intensively and to be able to fully develop the healing potential of pastoral care (Haußmann and Fritz 2021).

In addition, there are also ethical conflicts rooted in the dual affiliation and role. A professional ethic of hospital chaplaincy therefore mainly has the task of reflecting on this dual role and dealing with conflicts in this regard (Haußmann and Moos 2025). A blanket identification with the patient's will alone, or with the health goals or one's own religious convictions, is more likely to lead to intensified problems, as is currently the case with the discussion about assisted suicide (Coors and Farr 2022).

2.4 Challenges and Potentials of Outpatient-Care

In my work as a therapist, I (and most others in the team) found it extremely difficult and unsatisfying to organize good care for mind, body and soul in an outpatient setting. In inpatient settings, therapeutic work with patients is highly organized and team-oriented. In outpatient-settings, however, it is time-consuming and resource-intensive to collaborate with psychiatrists (to discuss medication), with insurances (to keep up therapy) and social institutions (e.g., youth welfare office, counselling centres for families to ensure therapeutic success in all areas of life and help with more support where needed). But although I am a theologian and deeply rooted in the structures and routines of religious and congregational life, it proved to be most difficult for the patients to find some contact or opportunities within the local church structures and communities with the aim to increase their social contacts or to find spiritual and religious resources. Although many patients would name religious issues, resources, or struggles, I almost never encountered a situation where I thought about interacting with a pastoral caregiver. Sometimes simply because of confidentiality issues as a therapist, but also because only few patients were rooted in a certain faith community.

When I organized a conference in Munich on the dialogue between cognitive behavioural psychotherapy and pastoral care, I found out that this was indeed one of the main open questions (Haußmann and Höfelschweiger 2020). How can an interprofessional exchange about specific cases or patients be facilitated without compromising confidentiality? Apparently, both the pastoral caregivers and the therapists felt that there were often religious questions or topics, and a cooperation was considered to be very interesting and fruitful by both sides. But it was completely unclear how this could be implemented in practice. While from the pastoral side there were concerns about pastoral confidentiality and therapists also were uncertain how to cooperate while upholding confidentiality, organizational questions predominated, such as: Who is responsible? Whom can I address from other professional backgrounds? How can I find out about patients who could benefit from networking between the healthcare system and church (congregations) – and how could they be supported beyond the boundaries of their professional disciplines? And what could spiritual care look like for individuals who want to, and should, decide who supports them, and how?

There is a lot of potential for outpatient care also in respect to digitalization. Whereas healthcare chaplaincy is usually perceived as bound to the interpersonal encounter in bodily presence, digital developments offer the possibility to communicate across space and time. Although there still is a lot of doubt and reserve from chaplains themselves, some already discovered the potential of digital presence as an advantage for their work (Winiger 2023; Swift 2020). Especially in outpatient settings, further contacts with pastoral and spiritual care would be possible. There are current developments working on platforms for digital communication in pastoral care and counselling that could also become very helpful in health care settings (Blackstein 2023).

As Gärtner (2022) pointed out, there is potential for hospital chaplains to act as communicators between different actors in the healthcare system. He refers to their role as “verticalists” in communicating and collaborating with other professionals and structures to ensure the patients’ all-encompassing health and healing (Gärtner 2022). For the inpatient setting, this may be already reality in some places – but what about outpatient settings? The following short case study may illustrate, how this could happen in outpatient healthcare practice.

2.5 Case Study: Joint Team Efforts to Find a Religious Caring Community

In our ward we once had patient who suffered from problems with concentration, low appetite, strong headaches and low motivation in continuing his daily life and his hobby as an artist. The diagnosis was long unclear. First, it was assumed that he showed early signs of dementia, which related to his problems with concentration and the loss of interests. The art therapist said it was unlikely that he really was a hobby artist once, since he was only drawing small circles with charcoal and pencil. Further along in the therapeutic process, it became clear in our sessions that he once painted huge canvases with bright and beautiful colours and He saw himself as a very religious person, but none of the staff had noticed so far.

At one time, we discussed his case in the weekly staff meeting and talked about him leaving the clinic soon. We wondered where he could find companionship and people who cared about him, I brought up the idea of contacting the local church congregation, since it occurred to me that his faith could be a resource. Since the hospital chaplain responsible for our clinic was very busy with seven wards at our clinic and 14 more at another clinic, it was impossible for her to attend every ward team meeting, and thus she relied on direct referral. The psychiatrist in charge contacted her, and she in turn contacted the church congregation and their pastor. We were able to find a group of older people interested in art where he could participate and finally found new friends sharing his love for art and religion.

When he left the hospital, he gave me one of his last paintings as a present: an abstract crucifixion scene in bright blue, purple and green colours, representing his vitality and regained love for life.

3 Evidence-Based Chaplaincy

Despite the important role of hospital chaplaincy for patients and healthcare workers (Haußmann and Fritz 2021; Roser 2021; Peng-Keller 2021) and the relevance of spirituality and religiosity to health (e.g. Balboni et al. 2022; Pargament 1997; Koenig 2012), there is very little empirical research on the effectiveness and activity of hospital chaplaincy and healthcare chaplaincy in Germany so far. Although the training and certification of hospital chaplains is based on quality standards (e.g. German Association for Pastoral Psychology, DGfP), fundamental research is only just beginning. However, from a patient-oriented perspective, the addressing of spiritual needs is highly important. In Denmark, over 80% of the patients reported strong spiritual needs (Stripp 2023), and similar observations exist in a German context (Büssing 2021). As secularization proceeds, reflections on the role of healthcare chaplains need to be extended in a contextual sensitive manner and according to the ability to address spirituality and meaning in a broad way yet also stay grounded in its own spiritual roots (cf. the contributions from Denmark, the Netherlands and the UK).

The reluctance to conduct outcome studies for chaplaincy in Germany can be traced back to methodological difficulties and theological questions, which in turn have historical roots (Fischer 2021; Karle 2010): how can pastoral action and spirituality be measured? At what point can one speak of a successful pastoral interaction? Can pastoral care, according to its basic understanding, be recorded in an evidence-based way at all, or should we even be afraid that pastoral care will be instrumentalized in health care?

Some scholars highlight, from a theological perspective, that pastoral care and spirituality are complex, partly unavailable processes that exceed the functional operationalization of quality control (Drechsel 2016). Thus, pastoral care above all would be characterized by unintentionality since it is not directed towards a certain goal. But most certainly, there are effects and also mentioned goals, starting with the idea of simply being there (Nolan 2011), and an attentive listening that does not aim at measurable change and optimization – despite the possibility to measure the outcomes with psychological or sociological instruments (for example with assessment tools or interviews). This is highlighted as the healing potential of spiritual care in the midst of the effect- and success-oriented logic of the hospital context. While the actors of healthcare are under permanent pressure to provide the best possible quality and are bound by professionally set goals for the contribution to healing, it is possible for hospital chaplains to endure the unchangeable and suboptimal situation together with the patient (Fischer 2021; Roser 2017). The solidarity in the face of an anthropological vulnerability that is acknowledged and even seen as the possibility of feeling and compassion is perceived as a strength of chaplaincy, and therefore also effective in a theological sense.

But pastoral and spiritual care are embedded in cognitive, affective and social behaviour and imprints and can be shaped accordingly. On this level of possibility lies the responsibility of every profession to be able to account for the reasons, goals and effects of its own actions. In order to be able to claim professionalism and healing effects, hospital chaplaincy must be examined for its nature, quality and results. However, a substantial body of international research and conceptual thinking exists on outcome-oriented pastoral care (Damen et al. 2020; Peery 2020). This requires a basic orientation towards the needs of others: to what extent is spiritual care appropriate, necessary and helpful for those receiving it? Also, an impact orientation is needed that corresponds to the ambivalent perspective on pastoral care. The following quote refers to that: "spirituality does not bear the stamp of success, although church pastoral care must reflect the effects of its actions in quality efforts" (Fischer 2021, 97, translation AH). Hospital chaplaincy is precisely "free of purpose and yet measurable" (Kohli Reichenbach 2018, translation AH). The research of Traugott Roser and his team has proven to be groundbreaking regarding the efficacy of healthcare chaplaincy. Nika Höfler has been able to show in a methodologically challenging but very profound study that vulnerability can function as a core category of hospital pastoral care (Höfler 2022, cf. the contribution by Roser). Therefore, these results contribute to an understanding of hospital chaplaincy not only in terms and logics of the healthcare system but also lead to a deep theological and anthropological differentiation of health and healing, holding on to the fragility, yet also the sensibility of human beings. However, the measurements cannot be borrowed from other disciplines; they have to be constructed due to the specific character of pastoral care in concept and practice.

The example in vignette B given above is a good illustration of the vulnerability of chaplaincy to the individual views of senior practitioners and managers. Whereas one of them might support chaplaincy – as in vignette B – others might not be convinced that chaplaincy offers a valuable perspective to patients. If further studies could highlight the evidence-based presence of chaplaincy rather than a presence supported by senior staff understanding, this might be politically smart.

Ultimately, the empirical measurement of effectiveness also may bring relief: on the one side, the chaplains' options for action are expanded and a general understanding of successful pastoral action is strengthened. On the other side, the review of the healthcare chaplaincy also strengthens the entire organization of the hospital context (Haußmann and Fritz 2022), whose various actors can complement and coordinate with each other through empirically reviewed quality standards (Fischer 2021). It can be assumed that the effects of pastoral care are not limited to the patients, but also positively influence the doctors' actions and the interprofessional collaboration between pastoral care providers and other professional groups (Lammer 2019). Interprofessional work in a team is one of the basic competences of pastoral caregivers. They network with other professional groups and, due to their freely allocatable time and their location between the systems of church and clinic, are largely independent to devote themselves to the team and the patients as needed. Because they are not identified with the healthcare system alone, they have a complementary perspective both in terms of anthropology (e.g., understanding of health and illness) and in terms of their assessment of processes in the system (e.g., in the ethical evaluation and assessment of situations; Roser 2017). This requires a basic ability to engage in dialogue and communication that is oriented towards other professions, but also able to understand other cultural and religious backgrounds. This is especially true for the Muslim (hospital) chaplaincy currently developing in Germany (Badawia, Erdem, and Abdallah 2020). So far, the education in pastoral care in Germany is mainly concentrated on theologians and pastors, and interaction with other professionals is rare. It would be an enormous benefit for pastoral care education to more closely embed the perspective of other professionals, but also to challenge them, as the encounter with the Other always is both an opportunity and uncomfortable at the same time (Doehring 2015).

From my practical experience as a psychotherapist in a clinical context, I want to add one more thought on the role of chaplains and their contribution to the healing process. As Traugott Roser (2017) has pointed out in his work on spiritual care, chaplaincy offers heterotopy and heterochrony in pointing to a transcendent reality out of this world (cf. the contribution of Traugott Roser). Many of my patients had contact and regular meetings with the healthcare chaplain at the clinic. When they were talking about what those meetings meant for them, they would say that they would just talk as "ordinary people", getting a coffee or going for a walk outside. It was a relief for them to interact outside the clinical context, not being seen as an ill patient who needs therapy, not to work on their health issues for a moment. In this way, the chaplain functions as a representation of the "normal", who brings the outside world beyond clinical context with him to some extent and addresses people in their humanity, their wholeness – despite their current health problems. In this way, healthcare chaplains contribute to healing because patients can feel like normal, healthy people who take time out of the context of their illness for a moment. Of course, chaplains would also be addressable for any religious issues, problems in the therapeutic or medical process, serving as a safe space for any topics. Cicely Saunders called the volunteering hospital caregivers the "experts of the everyday life", pointing to the importance of volunteers in hospital chaplaincy – which is another important current development in Germany to discuss. Since there is a lot of effort to increase the involvement of volunteers in hospital chaplaincy due to staff reduction of professional hospital chaplains, the danger of deprofessionalization in healthcare chaplaincy has to be taken into account. This points to the importance of a good education of those volunteers and their regular and case-based supervision by professional chaplains.

4 The Spirituality of Chaplains and Professional Self-Reflection

This issue is very interesting and important for (healthcare) chaplaincy, yet a very neglected area in terms of current research and theory. I have been addressing this in my research over the last few years, including empirical studies and theoretical reflection. To reverse the perspective for a starting point, the quotation from a trauma psychotherapist in Berlin points out the importance of spirituality for the perceived role of the chaplain:

> I think you as theologians have something at hand that we as psychologists and we as medical doctors don't have. You have faith and you have a Christian message. And that is actually what holds you up. [. . .] I think that is a strength of pastoral care that I don't have. And that also gives quite a lot to people (in Lammer 2019, 273 translation AH).

From the external perspective of the therapist, spirituality and spiritual practice are seen as a unique selling point of chaplaincy. Faith and the Christian message may add something new and unique to the healthcare system that supports and gives strength. As mentioned above, the research on religion/spirituality and health largely supports that idea. But so far, only few studies from the professional context of chaplaincy tell us something about the caregiver's spirituality and how this personal level of their faith and spiritual practice contributes to professional spiritual care.

In our study on pastoral care during the Covid-19 pandemic, we explored the spirituality of pastoral caregivers and its potential to support spiritual care and the coping with the pandemic (Haußmann 2022). Corresponding with the previous findings in literature about the interaction between spirituality and coping (Pargament 1997), it was found that spirituality served as a stabilizing effect and as a resource in times of stress. High centrality of religion and high daily spiritual experience correlated negatively with work distress. Despite the relatively low level of spiritual "dryness" (Büssing et al. 2013), some evidence seems to support the hypothesis that chaplains experiencing problems in their spirituality, e.g. a distant or absent God, religious doubts or resentment, would also be more sensitive to those feelings or experiences in their spiritual care practice. However, pastoral caregivers reporting those feelings reported more of those experiences in their spiritual care encounters (Haußmann 2022). In another study with pastoral caregivers from Switzerland and Germany during the pandemic, we found positive main effects of general religiosity on psychological burden and wellbeing, mediated by emotional competencies and spiritual struggles (Klein et al. 2024). The caregiver's spirituality can thus be interpreted as a resource in times of crisis and distress to ensure the maintenance of spiritual care.

But despite all evidence that spirituality of professional pastoral caregivers may serve as a coping resource, supporting spiritual care, it is also fair to say that – again corresponding with previous research on spirituality/religion and coping – it largely depends on the current situation and the content of spirituality itself, whether it is helpful or harmful in terms of coping. Spiritual struggles on the other hand (Exline 2013; Kenneth I Pargament and Exline 2022) are relevant to consider as well, especially since most professional spiritual caregivers are themselves highly religious. Thus, problems in the spiritual area have much more impact due to their higher centrality in the individuals' orienting system (Huber and Huber 2012).

Therefore, it seems reasonable to think about how to support chaplains in their spirituality and spiritual practice: embedding it more in education and training (although it is already part of some courses of CPE), discussing it on a theological level, and finding ways to enable spiritual practice (this is particularly relevant, as most pastors report having little or not enough time to practice their own spirituality, Winkelmann 2019; von Heyl 2003). Recent studies have pointed out the importance of a spiritual narrative of Christian chaplains that helps to form their identity and self-awareness of their marginalization in the healthcare system (according to the notion of "being alone") and the need of being recognized as providing helpful, yet also spiritual perspectives and practices for patients. Especially in the face of a rapidly changing world and ongoing secularization, pluralization and individualization, where more and more non-religious (e.g., humanist) chaplains offer spiritual care (cf. the contributions of Chris Swift and Wim Smeets), the role of Christian health care chaplaincy needs to be articulated clearly. At the same time, chaplains often face non-religious or religion-critical persons; thus, they need to be rooted in their own spiritual-religious tradition and at the same time be open to other worldviews, religions, and spiritualities. Pastoral care has always been open to all people; thus, a non-religious spiritual care is not necessarily the conclusion to be made – especially because everyone is rooted in their own worldview or framework of meaning; thus, there is also no neutral spirituality (cf. the contribution of Anne Vandenhoeck, this volume). However, chaplains need hermeneutic competence to be able to speak in different religious and spiritual contexts (Visser, Zock, and Muthert 2023) – yet also be aware of conflicting ideas of spirituality without fully adapting to the other's view (to become a "chameleon", to borrow Anne Vandenhoeck's expression) or by only finding similarities with another person (Visser, Zock, and Muthert 2023).

Looking at the theological literature in the German-speaking realm, however, it is noticeable that most publications on the subject are very presuppositional and normative (Haußmann 2023). Throughout, spirituality is seen by pastors as very positive and highly relevant for their professional performance, quite independent of its content. Connections between professionalism, personal faith and theological competence are rarely discussed explicitly and in detail. Yet, this seems to be precisely where an important interface and need for discussion lies. For example, considering the question of how much self-disclosure of one's own faith is appropriate in spiritual care, or if the care given should actually be about the faith of others. Or how theological reflection and personal experience relate to each other. Or where one actually learns to talk about one's own spiritual experiences in such a way that an exchange about them is also possible – when the sensitivity and vulnerability of this topic in particular is very high.

5 Current Developments and Outlook

Instead of discussing various paradigm changes, I would like to address some current important challenges that will affect healthcare chaplaincy in Germany, possibly also elsewhere, in the future. Some of these challenges are already being addressed, therefore an outlook on current developments in pastoral/spiritual care will be given concerning the regional church, education of pastoral care, and future research.

5.1 Outreaching Pastoral Care

I have been talking about the relevance of combining healthcare chaplaincy in outpatient and inpatient settings. An "outreaching" pastoral/spiritual care seems to be not only an important value and treasure of chaplaincy but could also serve as a more general orientation for healthcare chaplaincy. It seems to be one of the unique selling points of pastoral care compared to other healthcare services, which typically must be sought out by the person in need of help. Other than that, pastoral care also takes place in everyday encounters by reaching out to people in need (Mt 25,36: "I was sick and you cared for me"). But, as the hospital chaplain in vignette B also pointed out: that positive side of pastoral care not only takes a lot of time and effort, it is also challenging for the chaplain herself and additionally seems to conflict with an otherwise very desirable embeddedness in healthcare structures and processes.

Addressing the importance of an "outreaching" pastoral care, the protestant regional church in Baden seeks to extend their efforts towards greater networking between different healthcare and counselling services. This networking aims to intensify the communication between inpatient and outpatient healthcare. This also has to do with the increasing "outpatientization" of hospitals on the one hand, and with palliative care on the other. To this end, the regional synod has set up three temporary networking positions to structure and plan future developments. In this way, pastoral care in hospitals, retirement homes and hospices can be better networked and coordinated, but also in parishes and in outpatient services such as outpatient palliative care. The accompaniment of volunteers in pastoral care and visiting services should also be linked to this, ideally ecumenically. In this way, structures can be established that promote local communities of care.

5.2 Financing the Future of Healthcare Chaplaincy

At the same time, hospital chaplaincy in the regional church has to deal with 30% staff cutbacks, which affects all areas of church work and thus also health care chaplaincy. This is a step backwards, also because we know very well that people find the pastoral and diaconal activities of the church highly relevant (Bedford-Strohm and Jung 2015). Therefore, cutbacks in the area of pastoral care in hospitals, where there are many pastoral interactions and therefore much contact surface, are a problem. This is another reason why more networking with congregations and other psychosocial and medical services will be needed in the future in order to be able to maintain substantial and attainable pastoral care in hospitals at all. The involvement, training, and expansion of volunteers in pastoral care is therefore indispensable. We are currently conducting a study on voluntary work in pastoral care in Germany, about which very little is known so far empirically (Haußmann 2024). The aim of the study is to know more about the motives and experiences of pastoral caregivers in training and pastoral care practice so that we are able to continue to strengthen voluntary work in pastoral care and keep it attractive in the future.

On the one hand, volunteers in healthcare chaplaincy may be seen as a step towards deprofessionalization (Peng-Keller 2021). However, volunteers in healthcare chaplaincy still require guidance, support, and supervision from experts in the field, namely professionally educated healthcare chaplains. They would not only provide pastoral care themselves but also serve as mentors and supervisors for volunteers. This shift in their role and self-perception is crucial. Furthermore, volunteering in pastoral care should not take place without a pastoral care education of high quality (Haußmann 2024). Of course, the need for further professionalization of healthcare chaplaincy, driven by the ongoing differentiation of the healthcare system, is also required. Thus, a multifaceted approach – one that balances the need for professionalization with the need for adaptability and addressing pressing issues of structural and financial change – would seem the most promising.

Therefore, new models of financing healthcare chaplaincy must also be considered in the future. And for this, in turn, the argument for integrating hospital chaplaincy into the logics of the healthcare system is unavoidable. It also means expanding research on the effectiveness and outcomes of hospital chaplaincy.

References

Badawia, Tarek, Gülbahar Erdem, and Mahmoud Abdallah, eds. 2020. *Grundlagen muslimischer Seelsorge: Die muslimische Seele begreifen und versorgen*. Wiesbaden: Springer Fachmedien. https://doi.org/10.1007/978-3-658-29572-1.

Baden, Maximilian. 2020. 'Eine Entscheidung fürs Leben. Ausgewählte Ergebnisse einer Befragung zur Studienmotivation am Beginn des Theologiestudiums'. *Praktische Theologie* 55 (3): 167–75. https://doi.org/10.14315/prth-2020-550309.

Balboni, Tracy A, Tyler J Van der Weele, Stephanie D Doan-Soares, Katelyn NG Long, Betty R Ferrell, George Fitchett, Harold G Koenig, Paul A Bain, Christina Puchalski, and Karen E Steinhauser. 2022. 'Spirituality in Serious Illness and Health'. *Journal of the American Medical Association* 328 (2): 184–97.

Bedford-Strohm, Heinrich, and Volker Jung. 2015. *Vernetzte Vielfalt: Kirche angesichts von Individualisierung und Säkularisierung. Die fünfte EKD-Erhebung über Kirchenmitgliedschaft. Mit CD-ROM*. Gütersloh: Gütersloher Verlagshaus.

Blackstein, Achim. 2023. 'Das „Digitale Haus für Seelsorge und Beratung" entsteht'. *Spiritual Care* 12 (2): 156–59. https://doi.org/10.1515/spircare-2022-0056.

Büssing, Arndt, ed. 2021. *Spiritual Needs in Research and Practice: The Spiritual Needs Questionnaire as a Global Resource for Health and Social Care*. Cham: Springer International Publishing. https://doi.org/10.1007/978-3-030-70139-0.

Büssing, Arndt, Andreas Günther, Klaus Baumann, Eckhard Frick, and Christoph Jacobs. 2013. 'Spiritual Dryness as a Measure of a Specific Spiritual Crisis in Catholic Priests: Associations with Symptoms of Burnout and Distress'. *Evidence-Based Complementary and Alternative Medicine: eCAM* 2013:246797. https://doi.org/10.1155/2013/246797.

Coors, Michael, and Sebastian Farr, eds. 2022. *Seelsorge bei assistiertem Suizid: Ethik, Praktische Theologie und kirchliche Praxis*. Zürich: TVZ Theologischer Verlag Zürich.

Damen, Annelieke, Carmen Schumann, Carlo Leget, and George Fitchett. 2020. 'Can Outcome Research Respect the Integrity of Chaplaincy? A Review of Outcome Studies'. *Journal of Health Care Chaplaincy* 26 (4): 131–58. https://doi.org/10.1080/08854726.2019.1599258.

Doehring, Carrie. 2015. *The Practice of Pastoral Care: A Postmodern Approach*. Revised and Expanded edition. Louisville, Kentucky: Westminster John Knox Press.

Drechsel, Wolfgang. 2016. *Gemeindeseelsorge*. 2nd ed. Leipzig: Evangelische Verlagsanstalt.

Exline, Julie J, ed. 2013. 'Religious and Spiritual Struggles'. In *APA Handbook of Psychology, Religion, and Spirituality (Vol 1): Context, Theory, and Research*, 459–75. APA Handbooks in Psychology®. Washington, DC, US: American Psychological Association. https://doi.org/10.1037/14045-025.

Fischer, Michael. 2021. *Zukunft der Seelsorge im Gesundheitswesen: Zum Verständnis einer dynamischen Professionalität*. 1. Auflage. Würzburg: Echter Verlag.

Gärtner, Stefan. 2022. 'Seelsorgende als ‚Vertikalisten' im Krankenhaus'. *Spiritual Care* 11 (3): 284–87. https://doi.org/10.1515/spircare-2022-0023.

Haußmann, Annette. 2019. *'Ambivalenz und Dynamik. Eine empirische Studie zu Religion in der häuslichen Pflege.'* [Reihe: Praktische Theologie im Wissenschaftsdiskurs], Berlin/Boston 2019, https://doi.org/10.1515/9783110632880.

Haußmann, Annette. 2022. 'Spirituality of Professional Pastoral Caregivers during the Covid-19 Pandemic: Distress, Resources, and Consequences', November. https://doi.org/10.1163/15709256-20221433.

Haußmann, Annette. 2023. 'Spiritualität als Quelle einer vitalen Kirche? Pastoraltheologie und Kirchentheoretische Überlegungen'. In *'Wir können's ja nicht lassen . . .': Vitalität als Kennzeichen einer Kirche der Sendung.*, edited by F Eiffler and Reißmann, 93–116. Leipzig: Evangelische Verlagsanstalt.

Haußmann, Annette. 2024. 'Seelsorge – Auch im Ehrenamt!' In *Auf dem Weg zu einer seelsorglichen Kirche? Wissenschaftliche Auswertung der Bischöflichen Seelsorgevisitation in der Evangelischen Kirche in Mitteldeutschland (EKM) 2020–2024*, edited by Corinna Dahlgrün, 9:196–218. Studien Zur Theologie der Spiritualität. Linz: Arbeitsgemeinschaft Theologie der Spiritualität.

Haußmann, Annette, and Birthe Fritz. 2021. 'Was stärkt Seelsorge in Krisenzeiten?' *Pastoraltheologie* 110 (10): 397–415. https://doi.org/10.13109/path.2021.110.10.397.

Haußmann, Annette, and Birthe Fritz. 2022. 'Challenges for Pastoral Care in Times of Covid-19: Encounters, Contexts, Topics and Professional Needs – A Cross-Sectional Study'. *Health and Social Care Chaplaincy* 10 (2): 141–64. https://doi.org/10.1558/hscc.19554.

Haußmann, Annette, and Rainer Höfelschweiger. 2020. *Spiritualität und Sinn: Seelsorge und Kognitive Verhaltenstherapie im Dialog*. Leipzig: Evangelische Verlagsanstalt.

Haußmann, Annette and Thorsten Moos. 2025. „Verantwortete Seelsorge: Plädoyer für eine ethische Professionalisierung der Klinikseelsorge." In *Ethik in Seelsorge und Spiritual Care*, edited by Michael Coors, Sebastian Farr, Christof Mandry und Simon Peng-Keller, 59–94: De Gruyter. https://doi.org/10.1515/9783112219515-004

Heyl, Andreas von. 2003. *Zwischen Burnout und spiritueller Erneuerung*. Berlin: Peter Lang Group. https://www.peterlang.com/document/1096242.

Höfler, Nika. 2022. *Wirksamkeit von Krankenhausseelsorge: Eine qualitative Studie*. Arbeiten zur praktischen Theologie (APrTh) 88. Leipzig: Evangelische Verlagsanstalt. https://doi.org/10.5771/9783374072347.

Huber, Stefan, and Odilo W Huber. 2012. 'The Centrality of Religiosity Scale (CRS)'. *Religions* 3 (3): 710–24. https://doi.org/10.3390/rel3030710.

Karle, Isolde. 2010. 'Perspektiven der Krankenhausseelsorge'. *Wege zum Menschen* 62 (6): 537–55. https://doi.org/10.13109/weme.2010.62.6.537.

Klein, Constantin, Isabelle Noth, Annette Haußmann, and Hansjörg Znoj. 2024. 'Psychological Well-Being and Religiosity/Spirituality of Pastoral Caregivers in a Time of Crisis'. *Wege zum Menschen* 76 (1): 63–81. https://doi.org/10.13109/weme.2024.76.1.63.

Klessmann, Michael. 2019. 'Von der Krankenseelsorge zur Krankenhausseelsorge? Historische Streiflichter'. In *Handbuch der Krankenhausseelsorge*, 34–41. Vandenhoeck & Ruprecht. https://doi.org/10.13109/9783666616266.34.

Koenig, Harold G. 2012. 'Religion, Spirituality, and Health: The Research and Clinical Implications'. *ISRN Psychiatry* 2012 (December):1–33. https://doi.org/10.5402/2012/278730.

Kohli Reichenbach, Claudia. 2018. 'Krankenhausseelsorge im Fokus der Qualitätssicherung – Zweckfrei und doch messbar'. *Wege zum Menschen* 70 (4): 299–313. https://doi.org/10.13109/weme.2018.70.4.299.

Lammer, Kerstin. 2019. *Wie Seelsorge wirkt*. Stuttgart: W. Kohlhammer GmbH. https://doi.org/10.17433/978-3-17-036425-7.

Nolan, Steve. 2011. *Spiritual Care at the End of Life: The Chaplain as a 'Hopeful Presence'*. London: Jessica Kingsley Publishers.

Pargament, Kenneth I, and Julie J Exline. 2022. *Working with Spiritual Struggles in Psychotherapy: From Research to Practice*. New York: Guilford Publications.

Pargament, Kenneth I. 1997. *The Psychology of Religion and Coping: Theory, Research, Practice*. New York: Guilford Press.

Peery, Brent. 2020. *Outcome Oriented Chaplaincy: Perceptive, Intentional, and Effective Caring*. London and Philadelphia: Jessica Kingsley Publishers.

Peng-Keller, Simon. 2021. *Klinikseelsorge als spezialisierte Spiritual Care: Der christliche Heilungsauftrag im Horizont globaler Gesundheit*. Göttingen: Vandenhoeck & Ruprecht.

Roser, Traugott. 2017. *Spiritual Care: der Beitrag von Seelsorge zum Gesundheitswesen*. 2., Aktualisierte und erweiterte Auflage. Münchner Reihe palliative care, Band 3. Stuttgart: W. Kohlhammer.

Roser, Traugott. 2021. 'Den Dienst am Privaten leisten'. *Frankfurter Allgemeine Zeitung*, 26 January 2021.

Stripp, Tobias Anker. 2023. 'Religion and Spirituality in Contemporary Health Systems'. *Theology* 126 (5): 343–49. https://doi.org/10.1177/0040571X231194978.

Swift, Christopher. 2020. 'Being There, Virtually Being There, Being Absent: Chaplaincy in Social Care During the Covid-19 Pandemic'. *Health and Social Care Chaplaincy* 8 (2): 154–64. https://doi.org/10.1558/hscc.41870.

Visser, Anja, Hetty Zock, and Hanneke Muthert. 2023. 'Positioning Chaplaincy in the Pluralistic and Multidisciplinary Dutch Care Context'. *Religions* 14 (9): 1173. https://doi.org/10.3390/rel14091173.

Winiger, Fabian. 2023. 'The Changing Face of Spiritual Care: Current Developments in Telechaplaincy.' *Journal of Health Care Chaplaincy* 29 (1): 114–31. https://doi.org/10.1080/08854726.2022.2040895.

Winkelmann, Judith. 2019. *'Weil wir nicht vollkommen sein müssen': Zum Umgang mit Belastungen im Pfarrberuf*. Stuttgart: W. Kohlhammer GmbH. https://doi.org/10.17433/978-3-17-037059-3.

Chris Swift

Chaplaincy in a Time of Rapid Social Change

Abstract: The past thirty years have witnessed social and religious transformation at a pace which is unprecedented. In health care, this has led to a rapid diversification in the professional providers of spiritual care, ranging from an ever-increasing number of faiths to the emergence of provision by practitioners who are not religious. All of this reflects a decline in religious identification in the population at large, evidenced by national censuses. Drawing on a case study involving a Humanist chaplain and faith-identified colleagues, the challenges and opportunities of work in this new reality are discussed. The experience of using a more sensitive tool to capture complex patient religion/belief identity is described and explored. In considering this approach, it is recognised that a move away from simple (census-like) categories may produce information which has a) greater accuracy but also, b) contradictory and fragmentary data. Based on these discussions, proposals are made, relating to training; employers; and the provision of spiritual care to individuals and groups that are neurodiverse. Finally, theological consideration is given to Christian chaplaincy practice in the rapidly changing landscape of spirituality. In contexts of intensifying diversity and complexity, skilled and knowledgeable Christian chaplains have much to offer in helping people negotiate their beliefs within the experience of illness.

1 Background

The context in which health care chaplaincy operates in England has changed dramatically in the past century (Swift 2017). From a position in which the Church of England (CoE), as the Established Church, controlled almost all the key positions in chaplaincy, from lead roles in every hospital to national co-ordinating functions, chaplaincy has diversified at a remarkable rate. This change is linked to a decline in the influence of the CoE, alongside religious pluralisation and a decimation of Christian affiliation every decade (see the National Census for England and Wales, Office for National Statistics 2021). The largest growth in any category of belief has been in those stating 'none' or 'no religion' (Lee 2015). These

https://doi.org/10.1515/9783112205839-006

trends, while featuring some distinctive elements, are broadly similar to patterns discernible across the Western world.[1]

As late as the early 20th century, chaplains were significant figures in many hospitals, as well as in primary care. This was linked to historic roles in the allocation of resources, such as charities and 'alms houses'. Clergy often featured in the governance arrangements of public institutions, including hospitals. In 1948, with the founding of the UK's National Health Service (NHS), most clergy vanished from the governing bodies of hospitals. Effectively, chaplains became State employees. At the same time, as care no longer relied on charity, clergy influence in the provision of services in the community also diminished.

Possibly the single most significant watershed moment for chaplains after the founding of the NHS, was the election of the New Labour Government in 1997 (Swift 2017). This ushered in an era which saw much greater energy given to activities that promoted inclusion, diversity and equality. Chaplaincy was identified as an aspect of the health service which required reform to meet these priorities. For the first time ever, a Secretary of State for Health attended the launch of work which would initiate this reform and reflect the religious pluralism of the UK. At the time, the CoE was invited to lead on this work, alongside representatives of several world faiths.

The resulting work from this project was *Caring for the Spirit* (South Yorkshire Workforce Development Confederation 2003). This involved new policy guidance for the practice of chaplaincy and opened the door to much wider faith participation in paid positions in the NHS. There was aspiration to achieve a common data set and other elements of operation which would align chaplaincy more closely with the wider culture of the NHS. At the same time, this work sought to safeguard the religious identity of the chaplain and ensure that those working as chaplains continued to hold the active endorsement of their sending faith community.

In the following years, there was some discord about chaplaincy in England, arising from a tension between the CoE's determination to maintain control of chaplaincy, and chaplains' own aspirations to develop as a profession largely free from denominational interference. In 2015, the NHS in England published further guidance about chaplaincy and this made a significant change in opening positions to applications from humanist and non-religious practitioners (Swift 2015). This document was rooted strongly in equality legislation and values, which provided the outline of a legal framework for the appointment of chaplains as pub-

1 See also the chapters of Wim Smeets and Trace Haythorn in this volume.

licly funded health care staff. At the time of writing (2023) new guidance is expected.

Wendy Cadge (2013) has charted some of the ambiguities and opportunities for chaplains operating in a clinical context. While the traditional sources of authority for chaplains, ranging from Scripture to Church tradition and social deference, have waned, the ability to navigate the relationship of beliefs and medical practice continues to have value. In the case study set out below (created from authentic elements in three scenarios) the role of the chaplain is illustrated.

2 Spirituality and Neonatal Death – a Case Study

The average age of hospital patients (elderly) correlates with the demographic most likely to state religious affiliation. Consequently, a large teaching hospital in the north of England had done little to develop non-religious chaplaincy. There was no evidence of complaint from patients about the absence of a non-religious chaplain or pastoral carer on the team, or the availability of someone to speak with if needed. On the whole, religious chaplains felt comfortable having conversations with humanist and non-religious patients and staff. However, there was no information gathered as to how patients felt about pastoral care to non-religious patients being provided by religious chaplains. The chaplaincy manager began to identify a likely need for Humanist chaplaincy among younger adults, specifically in the delivery suite and neonatal care.

This need was identified because the hospital usually funded the arrangements for a funeral in the case of a neonatal death. Parents were often unconnected with a religious faith and had no residual link to a heritage of belief (e.g. through grandparents). Some articulated a defined position as non-religious, agnostic or atheist in their beliefs. This led to a situation in which Christian chaplains were meeting the non-religious needs of parents and families, for example, on occasions when broadly spiritual poems etc. were used, and in many respects the content was mainly non-religious.

To meet this perceived need a Humanist chaplaincy volunteer was recruited. Working closely with the chaplaincy manager during a period of induction, the Humanist volunteer was called on a number of times to support parents at the loss of a baby, and in the arrangements and conduct of the subsequent funerals. Two particular points of interest arose from this experience, which were shared in discussion with the chaplaincy manager.

- *At the time of loss there is limited scope for a discussion about appropriate words; texts; philosophical convictions; poetry etc. Experience of pastoral care*

suggests that only limited questioning should take place, but that families wish for something that relates to their experience and names the child.
- *During funeral preparations, the Humanist chaplain was sometimes offered texts to be read during the funeral, which included references to angels; heaven and other terms generally understood to be religious in character.*

The co-creation of secular liturgies, where the Humanist chaplain is a facilitator and guide, is seen as a positive dimension of non-religious care. The aim is to create something fitting and reflective of the person who has died, avoiding the imposition of religious ideas or images which are inauthentic to the beliefs of the deceased. However, at the point of death for an infant or baby, it would be pastorally inappropriate to engage in lengthy discussions or take the time to anything more than resources which might be immediately available. The parent, parents or family are typically in a state of shock and distress. Reflecting on this experience led the Humanist chaplain to engage with their national body to discuss whether some 'recommended' resources for this situation might be defined. However, care and attention to cultural diversity and individual belief would always be required.

In funeral preparation, when material appeared to include religious ideas, the Humanist chaplain would always check with the parent(s) whether they were certain they wanted a 'non-religious chaplain'. In every case, the parents affirmed that they would like the Humanist chaplain to officiate. The chaplain was very pragmatic in managing these requests and had no difficulty in using poetry that made reference to heaven; angels; or eventual reunion. In discussions, the Humanist chaplain and chaplaincy manager reflected on the different interpretations that can be attached to any given text. For example, what for a Christian might very clearly be 'the Lord's Prayer', could also be understood as a cultural artefact and an Aramaic poem of the first century CE. The Humanist chaplain did not feel required to know what parent(s) believed, so long as he was clear about his identity and role and that this was accepted.

3 Analysis

This brief case study provides considerable material for a discussion of chaplaincy, religion and non-religious spirituality in England in the twenty-first century. It alludes to the evolution of a form of Humanist chaplaincy which is developing its capacity to respond to the spiritual needs of non-religious people. Given the correlation of age and religious identification, it is likely that the greatest needs for non-religious spiritual care will arise among younger users of the health service. At the same time, this experience offers evidence that the nature of belief, or the ways in which texts are seen as helpful and comforting, is not clear-cut. The case study provides evidence that the nature of religious and spiritual conviction is shifting. In the mid-20th century, religious identity, knowledge and literacy was far greater than it is today. Many young people attended church services; confirmation classes; religious assemblies at school; and found Religious Education as a weekly class on the timetable. At a time when the UK population was considerably less diverse, a narrative of Christian belonging and belief was dominant. For people under the age of 40, this degree of contact with religious activities is considerably less than for those aged 50 and above.

In effect, we have moved from a situation where religious identity was fixed and defined to a much more fluid and eclectic set of beliefs. There are many ways in which this can be illustrated. In the research referred to below, while 55% of patients identified with some category of religious identify, 66% of all respondents stated that they prayed. This means that 11% of people who replied 'no religion' also said that they pray.

4 Religious (and Non-Religious) Identity

During 20 years working as a chaplain in the NHS, I began to encounter situations where the links to Christian faith, or knowledge about aspects of its practice, had become very tentative. For example, attending a situation of still-birth on the Delivery Suite – where a Christian chaplain had been requested out-of-hours – the grandmother of the baby and the mother spent a few moments trying to recall a much-loved prayer of the (now deceased): Grandmother: 'what was the prayer Nana really liked?' I was anticipating something along the lines of a 'Collect' or the poem 'Footprints'. Eventually, one of them said: 'O yes, it began "Our Father . . ."'. This highlighted to me the widening gap between Christian heritage and the knowledge of its practice.

In 2017, in a large Teaching Hospital in the north of England, a forty-question patient survey was administered to 316 patients by trained interviewers. During the process of developing the survey, it was recognised that traditional 'religion' questions do not reflect the reality that religious and non-religious identities may appear conflicting, dynamic or eclectic. The question used in national census and other surveys seems to reflect a way of religious identification characteristic of the 20th century, when there are examples of religious identity that are akin to factual and permanent characteristics. For example, in the First World War, British soldiers' identity tags typically included service number, surname and initials, regiment, sometimes battalion and rank – and religion (Imperial War Museums 2025).

The hospital-based survey took a different approach to this form of religious classification. Instead, the questionnaire used by interviewers began with an open question about whether the patient regarded themselves as having 'a religion, belief, philosophy of life, or spirituality'. If there was an affirmative response, a follow-up question asked the patient to describe their belief in their own words. A further inquiry asked the patient if they identified with any particular group within the community of belief which they identified in the earlier answer.

Allowing self-description, rather than a choice of pre-defined options, had a number of effects. It decreased the number of responses we would have expected to identify with a traditional religious category, when compared with the local census results. At the same time, it enabled people to have what would typically be interpreted as 'contradictory' identities, for example, that someone responding 'No' to Question 6 and 'Church of England' to question 7. People could nuance their replies, as happened when a few people said they were 'lapsed Church of England'. The value of this is that it is potentially a more accurate reflection of individual commitment. However, the research identified that 'spiritual' is an unclear concept for people and there was evidence of misunderstanding that equated this term with 'Spiritualism'. Overall, the research suggests that the traditional method of offering simple religious categories fails to do justice to the complexities of peoples' beliefs – but may be in the interests of religious leadership (by inflating the data). Equally, there is a tendency for Humanist and non-religious chaplains to claim representation for the growing number of patients who do not identify with any religion. This seems spurious, as most non-religious patients have provided no indication about how their beliefs might be supported. It also fails to account for the reality that people who state their religion as 'none' might still practice activities such as prayer. Furthermore, being no-religious does not automatically make someone a Humanist, as Humanism has more content than simply a conviction that there is no deity.

5 Implications for Specialised Spiritual Care

There is every indication that the 'non-aligned' – those who don't opt for a religious label – will continue to grow in the West. However, as the research and case study above imply, this does not mean that a hard category of non-religious belief exists in a doctrinal sense. The membership of belief orientated non-religious organisations remains small. People who do not associate with either a religious or Humanist identity may have complex, eclectic and seemingly contradictory convictions. These may also be highly dynamic rather than settled and established. As noted above, the term 'spiritual' can also be problematic in general conversation and lead to confusion of uncertainty.

I believe that this leads to a number of implications for specialized spiritual care:

1. All chaplains and pastoral workers should be trained to engage skilfully with pastoral conversations that are open to eclectic beliefs. There should be no judgementalism about the presence of these beliefs in someone's life. For example, a Humanist pastoral carer will need to recognise that elements of religious discourse (and even belief) may be present in patients who have identified as non-religious and who have selected to seek support from a Humanist. Equally, Christian chaplains with religious convictions will encounter people who believe in both the resurrection and reincarnation.
2. Hospital employers need to be educated about these shifting patterns, and how these may differ across the age demographic. Increasingly, this will see chaplains of different convictions engaged in supporting situations where families embody more than one religion or belief. Working skilfully together, chaplains must place the patient and carers at the centre of their professional focus and promote the best outcome for all concerned. This requires maturity, generosity and a shared understanding of spiritual health (Chris Swift, Handzo, and Cohen 2012).
3. Care must be taken to ensure that cognitive capacities are not privileged to the exclusion of all else. Sometimes, beliefs may appear to be contradictory due to conditions such as delirium and dementia. In some cases, the use of ritual and non-verbal means of connection will be the best response from the chaplain. This requires the chaplain gaining as much knowledge about the patient's beliefs as possible, but remaining open to the fact that these may have changed. It may also need the chaplain to explore with care and compassion different approaches in order to understand, iteratively, what is most supportive for the patient at the time of the intervention.

Central to how chaplains respond to these challenges is the ability to reflect intelligently on the experience of pastoral care in a changing society. The religious landscape in which I grew up is long gone, and the degree of awareness about religious language and how it is used has largely evaporated. This presents a challenge as we try to find new ways to express spiritual experiences and longings, as well as the risk of misunderstanding. I am not saying that these challenges did not exist before, but that there was a semi-orthodox framework in public life which enabled a way of communication that is now much more difficult to establish.

In a way similar to the creativity required in providing spiritual care during the restrictions of Covid-19, there is every indication that the future will require chaplains in the West to be creative, responsive and authentic. Having a mature and considered faith or belief system enables chaplains to engage with other spiritual idioms, and work across the complex world of religious literacy. There are still many fragments of Christian belief, culture and heritage largely hidden in the everyday languages and practices of the West. As these countries experience an incremental diversification in their populations, the capacity to work confidently and effectively with a range of spiritualities will enable the chaplain to negotiate the relationship of belief and health care in a way which benefits both institutions and individuals.

Communication is at the centre of how chaplains exercise their role. Too little work has been done about the detail and skill involved as chaplains 'curate' the spiritual experiences of people in their care. However, a very interesting and potentially promising avenue of research about chaplains' communication with patients emerged from the field of discourse analysis in a health care (Harvey et al. 2008). This arose from the analysis of a chaplain's interactions with patients, including the micro-details of pauses; silences and the chaplain's contribution to strengthening 'face' (a person's sense of positive social value). Unfortunately, this valuable initial work has not been developed further, which is a great pity as this effectively independent analysis of the chaplain's main occupational tool – conversation – revealed considerable skill, complexity and value. According to the researchers:

> With this quaint naivety the chaplain goes about his or her business using commonplace conversational devices such as the elicitation hooks identified here, which are deployed to facilitate the key spiritual activities of 'listening' and 'being with' the client. Hence there is significant value in demonstrating how this interaction is successfully achieved in language. (Harvey et al. 2008, 58)

This research makes clear that under the surface of skilled pastoral conversation, a delicate intervention is taking place that affirms the dignity of the patient while also enabling an open and frank account of the illness experience and its impact. There are a number of reasons why this might be happening. There is potentially advantage in the chaplain being seen as distinct from the purpose-orientated and outcome directed approach of most clinical interactions. Unlike almost everyone else working in the hospital, a chaplain might receive a patient referral without any significant indication of what the request is about. Consequently, the interaction between the chaplain and the patient is one in which purpose materialises, and where any action by the chaplain (e.g. prayer) appears during the course of the encounter. This openness, with its focus on emergent purpose, might serve as a caution – or qualification – of anything that drives the chaplain to identify purpose too quickly.

6 Faith Specificity, Generic Care and Reflective Practice

The diversification of chaplaincy in England has no doubt caused some anxiety in churches, which have been accustomed to providing religiously like-for-like care. However, this has only ever been achieved to a limited extent as churches are themselves diverse, and significantly different positions can be held within the same ecclesial community. A notable example of this would be the ordination of women in the Church of England. In reality, people in hospital will not always receive pastoral care from someone with identical convictions or the same church tradition (e.g. 'high church'). For this reason, it is not my view that diversification in the make-up of chaplaincy is to be resisted or undervalued. Hence, when I was involved in the periodic process to construct new NHS guidelines for chaplaincy (Swift 2015), it seemed both right and proper to more intentionally open the door to non-religious pastoral carers. Politically, this had the significant consequence that chaplaincy could no longer be criticised as exclusive State funding for religious practice. However, at the same time, this can cause practical difficulties given the tendency for out-of-hours calls to involve some expectation of religious rituals. For example, prayers at the end of life. There are neither the voluntary personnel nor the number of chaplains within teams to provide the diversity of available chaplains which may be required during a working day.

The reality is that all chaplains, of whatever faith or belief, are expected to have the skills necessary to provide generic pastoral and spiritual care. Conversations between people of different faith commitments can be illuminating and constructive. As the study of the chaplain's use of language makes clear, there are skills of narrative-elicitation that help people locate their experience creatively during a time of change. All chaplains can gain the skills needed to achieve this, even when the religio-cultural context of the patient is distinctly different from that of the chaplain. Respect, politeness and sensitive enquiry can all enable someone to find the language to give authentic expression to their experience. This is no small thing in health care, especially when the presence of the chaplain in the encounter may signal a broader sweep of meaning and purpose in which the patient's experience finds meaning.

For all these reasons, there is a priority for chaplains, both in formation and ongoing practice, to reflect – with careful attention to detail – on the experiences of pastoral encounter. Clinical Pastoral Education (CPE) has not been used systematically in the UK, but a recent initiative has seen the NHS give support to a pilot module. This approach offers a model of education that all chaplains can recognise, and which lays considerable emphasis on the detail of practice. For example, in the use of verbatims. Another approach piloted in England a few years ago saw a 24-hour residential event using specially trained medical actors to enable chaplains to focus on their pastoral practice and communication. Insights from the use of Objective Structured Clinical Examinations (OSCEs) were drawn on to evaluate the chaplains' performance and provide feedback. OSCEs were developed in 1975 and remain a commonly used method to assess competencies in communication across a range of clinical groups (Patrício et al. 2013). This focus on pastoral interaction has the potential to foster close working between chaplains of different beliefs and find common ground in the spiritual support of patients.

7 Theological Reflections on Christian Chaplaincy

During twenty years of work as a chaplain, I often reflected on my experiences of pastoral and spiritual care. Every situation felt unique, and many events in chaplaincy failed to fit into the traditional categories of religious practice. Rather like the tick-boxes of census enquiries about faith, the pastoral care boxes I'd been given in seminary seldom met the complex and blended realities of ministerial practice. At best, they had helped form a posture or way of being, which enabled creativity of care that responds to need as it is presented.

Theologically, this meant a lot of my spirituality and thinking was developed through praxis. For example, at times I found myself in situations where words offered very little and only some fragments of liturgy or Scripture seemed relevant. In the repeated exposure to these moments, I began to focus on my presence as a sign of 'the God who doesn't look away'. In the great theodicy of *Job*, it is something found in the initial response of the friends. Finding Job in such a state of suffering that words lacked the capacity to help, and cries of anguish were all the sound they could make. They echo Job's dishevelled state, tearing their clothes and throwing dust over themselves. They sit on the ground with him and because they can see that his suffering is beyond words, they remain silent for an extensive period of time.

In other words, although little might be transacted in terms of words or ritual, the request for a chaplain, and the chaplain's presence in a room, give a wordless witness that pain and sorrow are beheld. At moments when the life narrative of a family, including the implicit things we carry with us without much awareness of them (such as the idea life will be 'fair') collapses, the call and response of the chaplain hints at a small and unspoken belief that – beyond this chasm – there might be another side. I mean this both in the sense of 'heaven' (or some kind of eternal continuation) and also in the idea that a family derailed by tragedy might eventually find a new path which, at the moment, cannot be seen.

Some of the writing about chaplaincy might identify this as 'witnessing'. I'm not sure that fits entirely what I discern in this experience. It feels as though it is a decision, a commitment of will and spirit, not to cross to the other side of the road when grief approaches. There is no pleasure in beholding tragedy, but in the presence of the chaplain there may be a suggestion that while (for whatever reason) God does not swoop in to avert the suffering, neither does God vacate the experience. This may be a 'hope-against-hope' or an expression that the chaplain might carry, vicariously, a glimmer of a God the family cannot name, but will not wholly deny.

I have mentioned this approach to ministry as one which draws heavily on the concepts of being and presence. As I have written elsewhere (Swift 2020), in the light of the pandemic, 'being' is something found widely across a breadth of Anglophone literature about chaplaincy. However, this has not been followed up with many studies, perhaps because the theoretical idea is hard to study in operation. It would be helpful for the future of chaplaincy if more attention could be given to this and what it means for the recipients of pastoral care. At the moment, what little exists tends to see this practice through the eyes of the chaplain.

8 Theological Implications for Christian Chaplaincy

As noted above, chaplains now encounter less orthodox and more plural populations within health care facilities and services. There is little indication that this pace of change will abate. It is certainly important that further research is undertaken into chaplaincy practice, with particular attention to what takes place and how it is experienced. Some progress has been made on collecting and analysing case studies (Fitchett and Nolan 2015), and this is certainly a start. Other forms of research, including ethnography, have produced texts that can become the focus for professional analysis and reflection.

In considering the presence of the chaplain in the midst of devastating experiences, there is an appropriate link to be made with trauma theology. This is still a nascent field of study, and the research to date offers some understanding of what it means to be present before; during; and after a profound crisis. In related research the concept of 'moral injury' has also emerged and gained growing interest, not only in the military (Frame 2016), but in areas such as emergency departments in hospitals and in the wake of major disasters where choices are made that may go against the best practice a professional would wish to provide.

There is no doubt that the role of faith-specific chaplaincy (e.g. Christian, Muslim) relates to particular communities. It is unlikely that a Christian chaplain would be effective in ministering all the time to a Muslim community. This is not to say that there are moments when inter-faith encounters are without of merit. They are vital for sustaining understanding and peaceful coexistence. However, faith chaplains are skilled personnel who assist people by a form of listening and responding that recognises and values aspects of life which someone holds to be sacred within a recognisable framework of belief. In some cases, people may feel themselves to be only tenuously connected to the faith but expect the chaplain to understand how to mediate the beliefs they have in relation to the overall tradition. For example, the mother and grandmother of a baby asking the chaplain to say the prayer 'Nana always said'. After some struggling to recollect, they asked the chaplain if he knew the prayer beginning 'Our Father'. In many instances, people hold fragments of prayer, Bible passages or poetry which they look to the chaplain to contextualise and offer back to them.

For these reasons, if the Christian faith continues to decline in adherents, it is not clear what the role of a Christian chaplain would be. If faith-specific chaplaincy is to survive, it requires the presence within cared-for populations, such as a hospital, of people either loosely or closely connected with that faith. For this reason, the steep drop of people stating their faith as Christian in Western populations will make the public funding of faith-specific chaplaincy more open to question or, if funded and provided by churches, then it is likely that the resources available to send chaplains will become ever scarcer. While there is an elderly population, many of whom experienced several years of Christian faith formation in childhood, it is probable that the demand for Christian chaplaincy will continue for the next thirty years. Beyond that, it is possible that churches which persist within the overall direction of cultural change may still see care for the sick as a basic and essential act of service and witness. In this case, chaplaincy may continue as an external provision to institutions of care, where pastoral support is offered in the form of active listening etc. However, the use of ritual and faith explicit discussions may well diminish within this form of chaplaincy.

9 Conclusion

There is no doubt that the landscape of chaplaincy has become ever richer and more complex. I have written above about the social context of Western chaplaincy as well as its internal practices. As the range of traditions and beliefs engaged in chaplaincy has widened, the need for trusting and respectful working between chaplains of different convictions has become essential for the meaningful and effective operation of the service within a place of care. As the case study illustrates, this is perfectly possible when any sense of competition or doctrinal friction can be avoided. If the patient is placed at the heart of care, it is much more likely that chaplains can work creatively and constructively to find the most supportive approach. The weakening of the co-ordinating role of the CoE in chaplaincy has liberated the service to become more diverse; more imaginative; and more highly regarded in the NHS.

Focusing on the detail of pastoral work through reflective practice and CPE is probably one of the greatest drivers to both understanding what happens in spiritual care and for improving the way in which chaplains operate. There is great scope for theological development in the way Christian chaplains encounter health crises and support the spiritual needs of people receiving routine aspects of care. As research indicates, there is value in religious beliefs and practices as ways to promote healthy living. If this is the case, then supporting people when those beliefs come under strain is likely to increase the likelihood of those benefits persisting. For decades to come the role of the Christian chaplain, in many instances curating and interpreting vestigial religious memories and practices, will assist people in navigating the experiences of illness in the context of a fragmented and eclectic range of beliefs. The multi-faith and belief dynamics of many chaplaincies suggest that with a good degree of trust and confidence, the team as a whole can work to benefit recipients with wisdom, compassionate insight and a sensitivity. Within such teams, Christian chaplains will play a vital role both as religio-cultural advisers, but also as those continuing to provide direct care. We are now in a situation where neat boxes rarely contain people's beliefs and, consequently, chaplains need to be creative and authentic carers who work with patients so that those in receipt of care can find or continue a spirituality that sustains them during times of illness.

References

Cadge, Wendy. 2013. *Paging God: Religion in the Halls of Medicine*. First edition. Chicago; London: University of Chicago Press.

Fitchett, George, and Steve Nolan, eds. 2015. *Spiritual Care in Practice: Case Studies in Healthcare Chaplaincy*. London and Philadelphia: Jessica Kingsley Publishers.

Frame, Tom. 2016. *Moral Injury: Unseen Wounds in an Age of Barbarism*. Sydney, NSW: NewSouth.

Harvey, Kevin, Brian Brown, Paul Crawford, and Sally Candlin. 2008. '"Elicitation Hooks": A Discourse Analysis of Chaplain-Patient Interaction in Pastoral and Spiritual Care'. *The Journal of Pastoral Care & Counseling: JPCC* 62 (1–2): 43–61. https://doi.org/10.1177/154230500806200106.

Imperial War Museums. 2025. 'First World War Identity Tags'. First World War Identity Tags. 2025. https://www.iwm.org.uk/history/first-world-war-identity-tags.

Lee, Lois. 2015. *Recognizing the Non-Religious: Reimagining the Secular*. First edition. Oxford, United Kingdom: Oxford University Press.

Office for National Statistics. 2021. 'Religion, England and Wales: Census 2021'. 2021. https://www.ons.gov.uk/census/maps/choropleth/identity/religion/religion-tb/no-religion.

Patrício, Madalena Folque, Miguel Julião, Filipa Fareleira, and António Vaz Carneiro. 2013. 'Is the OSCE a Feasible Tool to Assess Competencies in Undergraduate Medical Education?' *Medical Teacher* 35 (6): 503–14. https://doi.org/10.3109/0142159X.2013.774330.

South Yorkshire Workforce Development Confederation. 2003. 'Caring for the Spirit: A Strategy for the Chaplaincy and Healthcare Workforce'. South Yorkshire Workforce Development Confederation.

Swift, Chris, George Handzo, and Jeffrey Cohen. 2012. 'Healthcare Chaplaincy'. In *Oxford Textbook of Spirituality in Healthcare*, edited by Mark R Cobb, Christina M Puchalski, and Bruce Rumbold, 185–90. Oxford, UK: Oxford University Press. https://doi.org/10.1093/med/9780199571390.003.0027.

Swift, Christopher. 2015. *NHS Chaplaincy Guidelines 2015: Promoting Excellence in Pastoral, Spiritual and Religious Care*. London: NHS England.

Swift, Christopher. 2017. *Hospital Chaplaincy in the Twenty-First Century: The Crisis of Spiritual Care on the NHS*. 2nd ed. London: Routledge. https://doi.org/10.4324/9781315253237.

Swift, Christopher. 2020. 'Being There, Virtually Being There, Being Absent: Chaplaincy in Social Care During the Covid-19 Pandemic'. *Health and Social Care Chaplaincy* 8 (2): 154–64. https://doi.org/10.1558/hscc.41870.

Trace Haythorn

“Tension Upon Tension Upon Tension”. The Complex Ecology of Christian Chaplains’ Service

Abstract: Christian healthcare chaplaincy has the potential to be a leading form of religious leadership in the twenty-first century; however, multiple tensions exist within and without the profession that hinder its impact and its self-understanding. In the following chapter, I will explore several of these tensions, striving to identify and, when possible, disentangle the complexities of chaplaincy practice, formation, and profession.

1 Introduction

Chaplaincy is having a moment. Since the initial lockdowns of the Covid-19 pandemic, stories about chaplains have appeared in a wide variety of newspapers, online media outlets, and television news segments. In many ways, it seems as if the world has made a new discovery, of these remarkable people who accompany people through their most vulnerable moments, sometimes into a new life, sometimes unto death. The stories often have an undertone of a question: “who would do such a thing?” And yet, chaplains have been serving in a variety of contexts for centuries.

These questions are not new to chaplains. One colleague shared attending a holiday party with her partner. While waiting in line for a drink, another party goer turned from a conversation, still slightly laughing, then after sharing names, asked, “And what do you do?” When she replied, “I’m a chaplain at the local hospital,” her new acquaintance grew quiet and simply replied with, “Oh.” End of conversation.

The role of chaplain requires a remarkable ability to adapt to multiple environments, expectations, and even practices in order to serve the constituency to which professional spiritual care providers are called. As employees of institutions, they serve as a part of a larger staff and can find themselves as either advocates for their organizations or voices of advocacy for the patients and families they serve. As members of faith traditions or other communities, they serve under the endorsement of those groups, though are often seen as something other than traditional clergy or lay leaders. As members of healthcare teams,

https://doi.org/10.1515/9783112205839-007

they serve alongside professionals who represent very different ways of understanding care. As the globe grows increasingly pluralistic and, in many cases, secularized, chaplains often find themselves navigating liminal spaces between their own convictions and the needs of vulnerable people at critical moments in their lives. And of course, there is the ever-present stereotype that chaplains are only around to deal with death and the aftermath. Tension upon tension upon tension.

In the US, such a response is complicated further by including "Christian" before "chaplain." Since the late 1970s, Christian has become a much more complex identity, as it has been identified with particular moral and political views. I have had some people blank when I identify as Christian, while others have wanted to grab my hands and pray together. At the same time, more and more faith traditions as well as humanists have adopted the title "chaplain" as one to describe those who offer professional spiritual care as representatives of their beliefs or values. This is all taking place during a rapid rise in the number of those who identify as "spiritual but not religious," a group disaffected with institutional religion but still longing for the kinds of spiritual practice and care that would seem to align beautifully with chaplains serving in pluralistic contexts. So, what does it mean for someone to claim the identity of "Christian chaplain" when both Christian and chaplain are contested terms, both embraced and rejected by different constituencies, and not always in ways that align clearly with familiar conventions or commonly held assumptions?

In many ways, I live at the intersection of many of the tensions embodied in this construct. I am a white, fifty-seven-year-old cisgender heterosexual man living in the southeastern United States. I am an ordained Presbyterian (USA) minister of word and sacrament, married to a Presbyterian (USA) minister of word and sacrament. I am the parent of two adult children, one who has a bachelor's degree from an elite private liberal arts college and the other who is in a college program for students with developmental disabilities. I have a Ph.D. in cultural foundations of education and am fascinated about how people make meaning and purpose in their lives, and I am a certified professional coach, serving alongside those seeking accompaniment and direction in their particular journeys. I was raised in Texas during the final days of school desegregation, and since leaving Texas in my early 20s I have lived in six states and another country. I have served as a chaplain in healthcare and in higher education, and as of this writing, I serve as the executive director and CEO of the largest accrediting body for clinical pastoral education in the US (if not the world). I am a co-founder of the Chaplaincy Innovation Lab, a member of the Transforming Chaplaincy Advisory Board, a faculty member of the George Washington Institute for Spirituality and Health (GWish) ISPEC curriculum, and a faculty member of the Intercultural Communication program of City of Hope Hospital in Los Angeles, CA.

I share this demographic information to situate myself within this larger conversation about chaplaincy. I enjoy a view of the field that has given me privileged access to conversations, visions, dreams, and fears within this profession. Most days I find myself positing that chaplaincy may within the next decade stand alongside congregational ministries in leading the religious lives of people around the world. Within the same hour, I will often find myself explaining yet again what chaplaincy and clinical pastoral education (CPE) are. And before the day ends, I will likely speak with someone who has experienced CPE as life-transforming, while someone else shares their deeply painful experience of an awful CPE unit.

If we are to discuss the tensions for Christian chaplains in healthcare, we have to recognize that the backdrop has all of these dimensions as well (and others I address later). We cannot understand the dynamics navigated by Christian chaplains without panning back to take into account the larger context in which they live, serve, and are formed. In the following pages, I will raise several such dynamics for your consideration.

2 The Dual Role of Chaplains

The question has been posed by our editors about the tension between the roles of chaplains as representatives of their particular faith tradition and the secular healthcare settings in which they serve. To address the question, we must take a step back and address the presumption, assumption and binary that inform its tension.

The presumption of the tension lies first in the question of the role and self-understanding of a Christian chaplain. What does the chaplain presume about themselves, about their role, about the context where they serve, and about the actors in that context (patients, families, clinicians, staff, etc.)? The assumption seems to be that the tension will be present and must be negotiated. To be clear, this depends entirely upon the (1) theological/meaning orientation the chaplain brings to the work and (2) the receptivity to that perspective by the context where the chaplain serves. This, of course, points to the binary that also seems implied in the question: matters of faith/meaning will necessarily be at odds with scientific, rational thinking. In many cases, however, these views are not oppositional in the traditional sense of religion vs. science; instead, the tension lies in the gods who are worshipped and the religious practices within both.

How, then, can a chaplain ground their practice(s) so that they are complementary – even essential – to the healthcare context? The vast majority of chaplains of all faiths/perspectives will identify "presence" as the essential character of what they offer in a healthcare setting. By presence, they do not presume to embody their understanding of the Divine. Nor do they reduce their rule to simply showing up, i.e., being present in the setting but not acting. Rather, the term presence refers to several specific characteristics of the chaplain and the role they play. Adams, in a review of the literature about presence, offers the following:

An operational definition of chaplain presence is establishing an environment of care based on empathy, curiosity, and respect in which the chaplain is attentive to the verbal and non-verbal two-way communication and assessing questions of the spiritual, the sacred, and of meaning providing concrete and appropriate psychosocial-spiritual interventions (Adams 2019).

Adam's definition assumes there is a spiritual dimension to human experience, one that needs particular care within the healthcare setting. There is nothing inherently antagonistic or oppositional to the secular setting. The art of presence practiced by an effective spiritual care provider makes the presence of the care recipient's source of meaning known and available as a part of the journey to spiritual health and well-being.[1] This journey is not one of doctrine but rather of compassion.

At its core, chaplaincy is the professional application of the spiritual dimensions of compassion. One would think that such a dynamic would be vital to wholistic healthcare. Grounding chaplaincy in compassion echoes the work of Karen Armstrong, who in February 2008 began a journey with faith leaders across a wide variety of faith groups to develop what is now the Charter for Compassion. In her scholarly research, Armstrong was delighted to learn how many of the world's great religions contained a scripture or saying that was a formulation of "The Golden Rule," i.e., do unto others as you would have them do unto you. Those committed to the Charter are now spread across over 440 cities and 54 countries.

The practical application of the spiritual dimensions of compassion in this vein describes the kind of presence chaplains offer those who are often facing the most vulnerable moments in their lives. For example, in a healthcare setting, the chaplain's role is to engage empathetically, recognizing the vulnerability of the other and offering the kind of care and concern that is most helpful to the patient. In so doing, the chaplain is enacting the spiritual dimensions of compassion, inviting the patient to draw upon their own spiritual resources.

1 For an overview of several definitions and studies of presence, see Kuis et al. (2015).

Unfortunately, too many Christian clergy and chaplains in the U.S.A. see their role as "winning souls for Jesus Christ," the active process of evangelizing and/or proselytizing. This presumptive practice holds that the chaplain has greater knowledge and understanding than the recipient of their "care," thus they must impart what they know in a manner they often perceive as similar to the work of clinicians. Most troubling is the self-understanding of their role as changing the faith perspectives of those who are often in some of the most vulnerable moments of their lives.

Rather than seeking to convert, chaplains are often the members of health care teams who help cultivate an appreciation for difference, providing resources to patients and staff alike. Should a patient find themselves at odds with a clinician, it is often a chaplain who serves as an advocate and/or mediator. "The Joint Commission recognizes the chaplain's advocacy role, referring to chaplains as "culture brokers." This competency reinforces the principle that it is never appropriate for chaplains to proselytize care recipients, further distinguishing professional chaplains from other spiritual providers" (Association of Professional Chaplains 2022).

My colleagues and I wrestled with the notion of what it means for chaplains to serve as cultural brokers, acknowledging the weight of such a term. In the US, brokers are often thought of within a financial context and tend to serve as go-betweens in relation to currency matters or stock trades. In using this term, our colleagues recognize the significance of the chaplain's role; it has substantive implications for whole person care. Traugott Roser made this point in our team conversations, noting the dual belonging of chaplains: we belong to a healthcare system as employees, and we belong to a faith tradition as ambassadors of a particular Christian tradition. The chaplain is often the member of the health care team who brings the context of the patient and their family to the larger care team, helping translate meaning, advocate for particular perspectives, and clarify reticence or hesitation based on religious beliefs. In many ways, the chaplain has a validating presence for the patient and for the medical context, belonging in part to both while also existing independent of both in many ways as well. It is in this context that we understand the chaplain as a "culture broker" (see Swinton, this volume).

Some Christian chaplains may balk at this definition as if it in some way waters down their vocation or their call: If they cannot bring people to Jesus, how can they in good conscience call themselves ministers of the Gospel? To those colleagues, I would remind them of the oft quoted words that are likely misattributed to St. Francis: "Preach the Gospel at all times, and when necessary, use words."

Of course, the response to this encouragement is often a concern about privileging works over faith. Many of my evangelical colleagues have concerns that people use quotes like these to avoid sharing their faith, feeling squeamish about talking so openly about something that can be so deeply personal. To be clear, chaplains have conversations about faith and belief all the time; they just don't use those conversations to try to persuade others to accept their view as the "right" or "correct" view. Daniel Nuzum raised this as a growing concern within his Irish context, where he is increasingly seen as an authority of the tradition they represent, even as chaplains often enjoy freedom from the constraints of their congregational colleagues because of the multi-faith context (Nuzum, this volume). Wim Smeets noted the complexity of chaplains' roles as both representing and belonging: representing a specific tradition while belonging to both a healthcare community as well as the faith community which they represent (Smeets, this volume). These tensions further reinforce the need for chaplains to develop their dexterity as cultural brokers, while also having a clear sense of themselves as they navigate these multiple commitments.

So much of effective chaplaincy is based on principles of getting out of our own way and working to be fully present to the patient (see earlier description of presence). Our task is to be so deeply grounded in our own understanding of the love of God we know in Jesus Christ that we can be open to whoever we meet, not as one ready to acquire a soul for Christ but as one who might offer the kind of compassion we see revealed in Jesus' life and witness. Only then can we help a patient access the spiritual resources already present within them, already available to them as a part of their journey towards healing and wholeness.

But even with this prohibition from these chaplaincy board certifying bodies in the US, healthcare providers carry their own concern about the role of chaplains in the care of patients. Physicians raise concerns that chaplains might lead a patient to reject certain forms of care due to religious beliefs, even when the physician sees that care as vital to a patient's wellness or healing. Others see chaplains as only having a role at the time of death (or after) but no relevance to daily well-being. In a study of ICU clinicians' attitudes towards chaplains, Choi et al. (2019) found only 38% of clinical fellows understood what chaplains do. As such, less than 10% of residents and fellows asked patients and families if they would like a visit from the chaplain. While Choi and his colleagues do not speculate as to why this may be the case, the underlying concerns clinicians may have and the lack of understanding clinicians have about chaplains' roles may fuel the ongoing tension between the roles.

To be fair to both healthcare chaplains and the contexts within which they serve, the larger societal and global messages about the roles of chaplains only seem to exacerbate understanding and valuing of chaplains' roles. For example, the World Health Organization sets forth the following assertions as a part of the preamble to its constitution:

- Health is a state of complete physical, mental and social well-being and not merely the absence of disease or infirmity.
- The enjoyment of the highest attainable standard of health is one of the fundamental rights of every human being without distinction of race, religion, political belief, economic or social condition.
- The health of all people is fundamental to the attainment of peace and security and is dependent on the fullest co-operation of individuals and States (World Health Organization 2025).

This definition is widely accepted by global health organizations such as the Centers for Disease Control (CDC) in the United States. While it is both elegant in its simplicity and highly functional in its brevity, the absence of "spiritual health" points to the tension in which healthcare chaplains serve. In their thorough analysis of religion in the WHO's efforts towards promoting global health, our colleagues Simon Peng-Keller, Fabian Winiger, and Raphael Rauch state, "While an impressive range of WHO documents highlights the importance of a 'spiritual dimension' in healthcare, the status of this dimension has remained fragile and marked by tensions. This is not least due to the fact that the WHO discourses we examined are only loosely linked, which indicates a partial lack of intraorganizational coordination and reception. It is particularly striking that the most important document, the 1984 resolution, has almost completely disappeared from the institutional memory of the WHO" (Peng-Keller, Winiger, and Rauch 2022, 200).

Of course, a change in the WHO's definition will not resolve this perceived tension. It is a binary that has been present in Western culture since the time of Galileo. The dualistic mindset of Western Enlightenment thought often poses frames of meaning against each other, positing that one must be right and the other wrong. It is less about better understanding and more about which side wins. One of the key tasks of chaplains is not to allow themselves to exacerbate this dynamic. That means chaplains must show up and interact with their clinical colleagues as valuable members of the healthcare team, as resources to the good work of their clinical colleagues, and as competent professionals who bring particular and valuable insights into the care of patients.

In many ways, this tension is a distraction from the vital care of patients. It is another place where our cultures displace their anxiety, frustration, fear, and pain. Perhaps chaplains can invite a new kind of transparency, honesty, and authenticity to bridge the gap rather than reinforcing an artificially constructed tension. As Michael Balboni noted, no one questions the role of the physician in the healthcare setting. At the same time, there is a tendency to silo the roles of each area – clinicians care for bodies, therapists and counsellors care for minds, and chaplains care for souls. Michael concludes by raising the powerful question: what if all of it is spiritual? (Balboni and Balboni, this volume).

3 A Question of Healing

The scene may be familiar to many: a preacher stands before a large auditorium while broadcasting far and wide. People with a wide variety of infirmities are lined up before him as he engages in a variety of actions meant to bring healing to those desperately seeking health, longing for something that can change their circumstances. And the audience/congregation is eventually introduced to the newly healed churchgoer. While the attention is often on the newly healed and the response of the attendees, who is this ultimately about? Is it about the healed, the witnesses, or the healer?

As I read the Gospels, spiritual healing is always multidimensional (Balboni et al. 2022). There is the healing of the individual – which comes ordinarily with no faith claims, no litmus tests for fidelity to God, no checklist of beliefs. Usually, the healed simply present themselves and their infirmity to Jesus (or later to the disciples) and return to their community, which is a key part of the story that is often overlooked. Many of these people would have been ostracized, alienated, or encamped away from the general population. Healing allows them to return to the fullness of community: to economic participation, religious rituals, civic engagement, and social interactions with friends and loved ones (and probably enemies as well). Quite simply, it transforms the whole of their existence, so much more than their physical difference(s).

Spiritual healing is a kind of "realignment" of meaning and community. When spiritual healing takes place, it often makes social, emotional, and even physical healing possible. It is a way of bringing heart, mind, and soul back in sync with God and God's purposes for human life. At the same time, spiritual healing does not necessarily imply physical healing. Instead, spiritual healing comes when the one who is healed is able to integrate their experience of illness fundamentally differently. Perspectives move beyond cause and effect to a more fully integrated view not only of the illness but of the person and their life.

4 Case Study

In many ways, this is the work of the chaplain, and a healthcare institution can make it possible through providing space and support for chaplains to do their work. In the early days of the AIDS/HIV crisis, I served as a chaplain in a general hospital in a northeastern US city. One of the patients, a gay man in his early 20s, was near end-stage AIDS, with lesions on his brain that were rapidly deteriorating his ability to communicate. He asked that his parents be notified, then added that they had been estranged for several years. He explained that they had great difficulty with his love for a man, grounding their argument in their Baptist faith. When they arrived, they brought threats of legal action to prevent the patient's partner from visiting. The parents were grieving their son even as they shamed him. It was an incredibly painful experience for all involved.

The patient requested that he wanted hospice care and wanted to die at home. His parents saw an opportunity to further restrict the partner by bringing their son to their home. The healthcare team decided I could play a vital role in the spiritual healing of all involved. Working closely with the social worker, we engaged the parents' fear and sadness. We met with the partner and the patient to be clear about their wishes. Those wishes including making sure the son could return to the home he shared with his partner, a decision that further angered his parents. I often prayed with the parents, though the father often needed to add to my prayers. When it became clear the young man had only days to live, something shifted in the parents. They asked if they could visit their son's home. The partner made them dinner, and the partner's mother joined them for the meal. By the end of the meal, the parents agreed to allow their son to return to his home with his partner. They clarified their hopes in spending time with him in his last days. When the dishes were cleared, all parties had come to an agreement about how things would proceed in the coming days.

To be clear, this was not a happily ever after story. There was still great pain at many levels. But the shift was a kind of spiritual healing, for it brought some comfort to the patient, his partner, and his parents. The community was changed through powers far greater than any of us who made this journey with them. What once seemed impossible became real. And much like physical healing, there was plenty of work (and healing) for everyone to do long after the patient died. But it was clear that many significant shifts had taken place within and between everyone involved. Those shifts were "God spaces," the places where the Spirit invited life amidst so many layers of death.

For chaplains, it is often this kind of "faithful facilitation" that makes room for spiritual healing. It would be hubris to claim my role in this particular case as having been a spiritual healer. I was a witness to the healing that took place through the loving and faithful actions of so many. It wasn't perfect. And it often didn't feel good. But the man died surrounded by the love that had carried him through life.

5 Personal Spiritual Practice and Professionalism

Decades ago, Clinical Pastoral Education programs (CPE) were run by Christian denominations, seminaries, or institutions. Students from the same tradition could gather and explore best practices for spiritual care, while also identifying the central theological tenets undergirding those practices. Some of these programs were additions to seminaries, working in close conversation with pastoral care departments, denominational judicatures (when relevant), and field education offices.

Over time, CPE groups grew increasingly diverse, as did the seminary campuses from which the students came. Supervisors placed less and less emphasis on pastoral theology and more on psychology, sociology, and topics related to healthcare. Departments developed new names, like "spiritual care" and "spiritual health," both indicators of the growing diversity both within the field and in the populations people were called to serve. As a part of a recent restructuring of accreditation standards within the Association of Theological Schools (ATS), students can now complete a Master of Divinity (M.Div.) degree without having taken even a basic course in spiritual care. At the same time, fewer and fewer students are coming into CPE with M.Divs., preferring two-year degrees or equivalencies, raising many questions about how a chaplain will be formed, will practice, and will be theologically grounded.

Ideally, a CPE program helps a student deepen their self-understanding and core convictions, helping them grow into a space where the beliefs and convictions of others are seen as resources for those others, not threats or challenges to the chaplain. It is from such a place and perspective that the chaplaincy with the greatest integrity emerges. This is not to in any way disparage the rich learning that continues to take place in both seminaries and CPE. To the contrary, many CPE programs now help students develop specializations in particular fields within healthcare, like palliative care, oncology, or pediatrics. CPE supervisors/educators often build their programs so that students can become richly conversant with theories like family systems theory or internal family systems. More and more leaders are paying attention to the important developments taking place in neuroscience, helping students become more aware of their bodies and the ways bodies interact at the neural level (as described in polyvagal theory, for example). This has led to significant improvements in the ways chaplains care for people who have suffered great trauma or moral injury. Many leaders involved in this process, however, have raised important questions about where and how the theological formation and grounding takes place for students.

Many seminaries in the US have offered spiritual direction for students as a way to address this formation gap. Ideally, every student would have access to the kinds of developmental opportunities a spiritual director could facilitate while learning the art of chaplaincy. Weekly sessions for students engaged in their first unit would be ideal, while students participating in year-long programs may find bi-weekly or monthly sessions more effective, allowing more time for integration and reflection.

Once a chaplain is employed by a healthcare institution, the impetus for ongoing integration and reflection usually falls on the chaplain to seek. Even among those who are board certified, there is little guidance or supervision available to those who seek to deepen their own faith while working to nurture others. As our societies become increasingly pluralistic, this may be one of the most significant areas that needs attention to advance the integrity of the profession. What if spiritual direction was included as an integral component of every CPE unit, thus allowing students to not simply engage in process and content, but also to deepen their particular faith in ways that allows them to more effectively serve all people regardless of how they ground their personal meaning and purpose?

6 Paradigm Shift within CPE?

Healthcare has entered an age that historians may one day identify as the "age of measurement." In many ways, this age has much promise. The aggregation and analysis of data can lead to important breakthroughs in the ways care is provided, interventions are developed, and therapies are deployed. For decades, a small group of CPE educators and researchers have worked to identify kinds of measurement (the "how") and that which they could meaningfully measure (the "what") to demonstrate the efficacy of professional spiritual care. Because spiritual care is not considered a "revenue generating center" within hospitals, the increasing attention to healthcare costs has made such measurement more and more of an imperative if spiritual care departments are to have a future in the institutions they serve.

This emphasis has had a significant impact on CPE curricula in several ways. First, increasingly, CPE residencies teach research literacy so that chaplains can know how to read research and to assess it for its overall efficacy. Second, education for future CPE supervisors/educators now often includes requirements in research literacy, with specific standards and/or competencies included as a part of supervisory education. Third, ACPE has created a fund for spiritual care resource and grants up to $100,000 USD annually for research and/or innovations in CPE and professional spiritual care. While these funds are a far cry from the kinds of investments the John Templeton Foundation has made in spiritual care research, they do signal a shift in what the largest US accrediting body for CPE has established as a priority.

In many ways, the Templeton grant that led to the formation of Transforming Chaplaincy at Rush University Hospital marked the major shift within the profession, a turn from a few researchers engaging in this work towards a more systematic effort to establish research as a primary competency for healthcare chaplaincy. George Fitchett and Wendy Cadge, co-principal investigators on the grant, have continued to build on that work, George within Transforming Chaplaincy and Wendy through the Chaplaincy Innovation Lab housed at Brandeis University. These two entities have become vital resources in the US and abroad for the study of chaplaincy and for the efforts towards improving the quality of CPE programs across the US and abroad.

The systematic review published by Tracy Balboni, et al. (2022) in the Journal of the American Medical Association (JAMA) will serve as perhaps the most important benchmark in terms of the argument for evidence-based spiritual care. While some organizations and CPE programs have claimed to offer such evidence, this article is the first that provides substantive evidence of the efficacy of spiritual care for general health outcomes and for serious illness. The authors conclude the article stating:

"These suggested implications for serious illness and health outcomes could aid in furthering the National Academy of Medicine's goals for improving health care quality in the 21st century, calling for more attention to patients' values, often shaped by spiritual views, in health care. While research and ethical reflection is needed to determine their practical application in clinical and other health settings, these suggested implications suggest a potential to improve well-being for patients and other populations, including vulnerable groups and those with the highest burden of disease. Furthermore, potential implications may apply to a range of important outcomes including overall mortality, quality of life, mental health, and substance use. However, attention to matters of spirituality in health care should be individualized, patient-centered, and respectful of beliefs and preferences" (Balboni et al. 2022, 195).

The implications for CPE as well as hospital grand rounds and other educational opportunities are clear: CPE programs must teach students how to help integrate spirituality as a part of an institution's commitments to patient-centered care. It moves CPE and professional spirituality beyond having to defend their value and placing them at the heart of the care of patients by addressing and teaching others to recognize the fundamental questions of meaning they will likely encounter during hospitalization.

By its very nature, CPE has evolved since the earliest days of experimentation by Anton Boisen with his new method of adult learning. Because CPE is so focused on "process," it must inevitably evolve if it takes its learners seriously. At the same time, not all evolution comes from within the practices of CPE. There are forces beyond the healthcare settings where CPE is practiced that are contributing to what may be seen as a paradigm shift. In the summer of 2022, ACPE returned to the US Department of Education (USDE) for its five-year review. Having been recognized since the late 1960s, this was in many ways a routine visit. In many other ways, it marked a very different moment, one that, much like healthcare, signaled a new and challenging emphasis on student learning outcomes within CPE programs. Because the USDE primarily recognizes accreditors of higher education programs located within colleges and universities, there is a strong emphasis on having program accreditors like ACPE follow similar expectations and requirements. For example, ACPE has been asked to provide much more objective criteria for student learning, including timelines and measurements. This requirement follows the pattern within healthcare, seeking more and more quantitative data as the measures of learning, allowing ACPE, its programs, students and other stakeholders to more effectively compare the quality of the programs and student learning within them.

These changing are taking place within significant shifts within the larger culture as well. CPE began as a white, Protestant, and largely male enterprise. While it has grown increasingly diverse, the deep trenches of CPE's cultural memory have made steering the organization in new directions very difficult. Questions of racial discrimination, gender bias, and disregard of gender identity are the lived experiences of educators and students, along with the healthcare communities they serve. CPE supervisors and chaplains play vital roles in advocating for justice within these systems, but this work is extraordinarily difficult to measure. Because these efforts are also often antagonistic to healthcare administrators, they tend not to be valued in ways that advance programmatic goals, even though they are included in educational standards.

While the emphasis on outcomes within hospital settings and through government regulations have been a significant driver of the changes within CPE, it is arguable the changing nature and expectations of students is as strong if not stronger in terms of its effects on the shifting models of CPE. There are many stereotypes of Generations Y and Z, and I don't want to reinforce any of them. What we have seen within ACPE has been a rising demand for CPE to become more appreciative and less "deconstructive." For many years, students have grown to expect that CPE would involve a process that challenges their beliefs and assumptions, compels examinations of significant relationships (especially family), and drives them to push for clarity about their sense of self and their place in the world. Today, students are increasingly rejecting this approach to CPE, arguing instead for models that recognize that when they enter a program they come with gifts and talents, and they expect to build on those gifts and talents rather than focus on their perceived weaknesses and deficits. They also expect their educators to be understanding of (or at least curious about) the lived experiences the students bring into their CPE programs.

This shift among students means CPE supervisors must engage their work very differently than how they were trained. Because there is such varied preparation in spiritual care, educators cannot assume their students have even a basic understanding of the spiritual foundations of chaplaincy. Anne Vandenhoeck argued that Christian CPE educators need to reclaim the idea first proffered by Moltmann, that the essential tension for a Christian chaplain comes in living metaphorically on Holy Saturday, i.e. between the tension of Good Friday and Easter Sunday (Moltmann 2021).

In addition to introducing such theological foundations, CPE programs should explore models grounded in appreciative inquiry (Center for Appreciative Inquiry 2025). Such a shift will have multiple effects. First, students come to clinical pastoral education as adults; most of them have completed or are in the process of completing graduate degrees. They will each have their own complex histories, knowledge, biases, and gifts. Historically, some educators have seen these adult students as deconstruction projects, i.e., individuals to be broken down into their component parts and reassembled in ways that they might have greater understanding and be more effective in serving. This process ignores that most adult educational theory sees people essentially "formed" by their mid to late 20s, thus making their education process far more effective when it draws upon their existing knowledge, strengths, capacities, and competencies. Second, it approaches the processing of students' different theologies from the lens of asset rather than potentially problematic. Imagine a student wrestling with a question of theodicy. Another student offers a different perspective from their own tradition. How different would the discussion be if the supervisor invited the group to name the strengths of both positions, an exercise that will also facilitate the appreciative engagement of patients from different traditions? Third, CPE students are often emotionally, spiritually, and physically exhausted from their rapid immersion in such difficult work. If the students' strengths are engaged, the experience of the student will not only be deeper learning about their individual capacities and competencies, but also the utilization of those strengths to provide resiliency in the face of so much pain and grief in the healthcare setting. Fourth, if students learn to approach their peers as gifted and develop practices that help them integrate that approach, they are much more likely to do the same with those whom they will serve in their different ministries once they complete CPE and/or seminary.

Rarely do single factors lead to paradigm shifts. In the case of CPE, the expectation of "outcomes" within healthcare settings, the emergence of spiritual care research, the changing socio-cultural environment (especially the increasingly pluralistic contexts in which these programs function), and the significant change in the expectations of students about CPE have all contributed to this new day. As we are very much in the middle of it, it is incredibly difficult to say where all of this is leading. What is clear is that "trusting the process" will require significant learning and adaptation on the part of accreditors and educators in the coming years.

7 Conclusion

Historically, when so many forces find themselves in places of such tension, it is indicative of the kinds of paradigm shifts that lead to fundamentally new understandings of our human ways of being. We are a planet on the edge: on the edge of environmental devastation; racial, religious, gender, and ethnic transformation; economic restructuring; and global warfare, even unto nuclear proliferation. Healthcare sits at the intersection of all of these dynamics, and because of healthcare's role, Christian chaplains can expect to find themselves in increasing demand. To faithfully respond, we must collectively become much more aware of the tension-filled waters in which we live and serve, position ourselves as leaders of the transformations, and muster the courage and vision to become that which God has longed for all along.

References

Adams, Kevin. 2019. 'Defining and Operationalizing Chaplain Presence: A Review'. Journal of Religion and Health 58 (4): 1246–58. https://doi.org/10.1007/s10943-018-00746-x.

Association of Professional Chaplains. 2022. 'The Impact of Professional Spiritual Care'. https://www.professionalchaplains.org/Files/resources/The%20Impact%20of%20Professional%20Spiritual%20Care_PDF.pdf.

Balboni, Tracy A, Tyler J Van der Weele, Stephanie D Doan-Soares, Katelyn NG Long, Betty R Ferrell, George Fitchett, Harold G Koenig, Paul A Bain, Christina Puchalski, and Karen E Steinhauser.

2022. 'Spirituality in Serious Illness and Health'. Journal of the American Medical Association 328 (2): 184–97.
Center for Appreciative Inquiry. 2025. 'What Is Appreciative Inquiry?' 2025. https://www.centerforappreciativeinquiry.net/resources/what-is-appreciative-inquiry-ai/.
Choi, Philip J, Vinca Chow, Farr A Curlin, and Christopher E Cox. 2019. 'Intensive Care Clinicians' Views on the Role of Chaplains'. Journal of Health Care Chaplaincy 25 (3): 89–98. https://doi.org/10.1080/08854726.2018.1538438.
Kuis, Esther E, Anne Goossensen, Jolanda Van Dijke, and Andries J Baart. 2015. 'Self-report Questionnaire for Measuring Presence: Development and Initial Validation'. Scandinavian Journal of Caring Sciences 29 (1): 173–82. https://doi.org/10.1111/scs.12130.
Moltmann, Jürgen. 2021. Theology of Hope: For the 21st Century. London: SCM Press.
Peng-Keller, Simon, Fabian Winiger, and Raphael Rauch. 2022. The Spirit of Global Health: The World Health Organization and the 'Spiritual Dimension' of Health, 1946–2021. Oxford, New York: Oxford University Press.
World Health Organization. 2025. 'Constitution of the World Health Organization'. 2025. https://www.who.int/about/governance/constitution.

Daniel Nuzum

Spiritual Breadth and Breath. The Evolving Relationship between Christian Healthcare Chaplains, Faith Communities and Healthcare Institutions

Abstract: This chapter outlines the development of healthcare chaplaincy in Ireland from a primarily religious expression and provision towards a broader pluralistic approach. This development is traced alongside the changing demographics of Irish society and the growing recognition of the development of healthcare chaplaincy as a profession. The evolving dual relationship of the Christian healthcare chaplain to their faith community and to the healthcare institution is illustrated as a creative liminal space. Drawing on a case study of a baby diagnosed with a congenital fetal anomaly, the chapter illustrates how 'Christian healthcare chaplaincy' has much to contribute to professional spiritual care in a pluralist context. The contribution of Clinical Pastoral Education to the education and formation of healthcare chaplains/ spiritual carers is outlined. CPE in Ireland continues to develop as a competency-based approach with international reciprocity. The developments in CPE as an integrative process are congruent with developments in wider healthcare education and the scholarship of teaching and learning. These developments in practice, approach, and education recognize the importance of the spiritual identity of the healthcare chaplain and their place as the spiritual care expert on the interdisciplinary healthcare team.

1 Introduction

Joy* (fictitious name) was diagnosed with a life-limiting congenital anomaly during pregnancy. Prior to this diagnosis, her parents Mary and Christophe were planning for the arrival of their first baby with excitement. Their excitement was replaced by sadness, fear and unknowing, as the significance of this unwanted news became apparent. With each passing week and more detailed anatomy scans, the reality of loss was experienced in the 'here and now' and as an impending anticipated loss that was uncharted and unwelcome territory for Mary and Christophe. I was asked to see Mary and Christophe a few weeks after the diagnosis and accompanied them for the remaining ten weeks of their pregnancy.

https://doi.org/10.1515/9783112205839-008

I am a healthcare chaplain, and I entered my profession as someone who is an ordained Anglican Priest. I was appointed to my role following a recruitment process with my church and the hospital I work in. In addition to applying for a 'job' I also sensed a calling or vocation to serve in this distinctive way. I am a husband, a parent, a former nurse and someone who has experienced pregnancy loss, and therefore I sensed a natural pull towards perinatal ministry and specialized in this area – undergirded by pastoral experience, Clinical Pastoral Education (CPE) training and specialized perinatal bereavement and palliative care training. I have a dual relationship with both my church and the hospital: I am accountable to both in addition to being accountable to the profession of healthcare chaplaincy as an accredited healthcare chaplain and a CPE supervisor educator.

Joy's parents professed no particular faith. What had I therefore to offer them at this most difficult time in their young adult lives as they heard the unimaginable about their daughter? They would not want or welcome a church or religious approach to their loss and grief. They would most likely not want prayer, sacraments or religious ritual. What then can I bring to attend to and respond to their spiritual questions and needs? Can I with integrity provide the care they would wish for if that care were not what I would wish for myself? Can I offer care or a ritual that is not infused with the values of my faith and what I hold dear? To reflect on these issues is core to contemporary healthcare ministry and pastoral/spiritual care.

Joy's parents did not need my church, but they did have existential and spiritual distress and concern. They explored questions about meaning, value, the questions "why", "why us?" and "did we do something wrong?". They wrestled with conflicted emotions such as love, anger, fear, and hope with a searingly honest vulnerability and in a way they never had to do before. They cried, they consoled one another, they marvelled as they saw the details of Joy's fingers on the ultrasound scan. They experienced connection, love, tenderness, fear, and vulnerability; longing yet dreading the day of Joy's birth. Joy's mum captured this poignantly as she said, "every day closer to her birth is a day closer to her death". They yearned to say hello but knew this would inevitably be followed all too soon by a goodbye. They wrestled with the possibility of terminating their pregnancy, which met the strict diagnostic and prognostic threshold in accordance with recently introduced legislation in Ireland in 2019.

2 A Religious Response to Need

Health and illness have been intricately woven through the fabric of the story of faith in the Jewish and Christian traditions. Indeed, health and the lack of health, illness or dis-ease have carried the hermeneutical weight of the blessing or otherwise of God in the faith story and sacred texts of the Hebrew and Christian Scriptures. Recognising the importance of health and wellbeing as having both personal and communal/community dimensions has placed ministry and care to those who are ill, frail or struggling as important in the overall outworking or practice of faith for the Christian. There are many instances in Scripture where care of those who are ill is enjoined on the Christian community. This care had both a pastoral and salvific approach in the restoration to wholeness: *shalom*. Like many parts of the world, many of the earliest healthcare facilities in Ireland were established by religious communities, and most continue to this day. Many of these early religious foundations have evolved alongside civic society as modern healthcare facilities and centres of excellence have developed. In Ireland, this includes up to fifty per cent of our current public and larger acute hospitals and most of our specialist palliative care hospices, which can trace their history to a religious foundation. These developments have happened concurrently with the development of medicine, nursing and other healthcare professions.

Recognising the pastoral and often the practical needs of those who are ill led to the development of designated roles to provide for the religious and spiritual needs of patients. As with the provision of healthcare by faith communities as a response to immense need that was not addressed adequately by society, so too the provision of pastoral care was seen as an extension of the ministry of the faith community and was usually textured by the particular charism of the community or religious order. As medicine, science, technology, skill and innovation developed, healthcare institutions have evolved from being primarily religious institutions to what are now modern complex healthcare systems shaped by innovation, evidence-based practice, clinical skill and care, and cutting-edge research.

3 Healthcare, Faith and Chaplaincy in Ireland: An Evolving Reality

As healthcare developments took place since the foundation of the Irish state in 1922, faith communities and churches evolved from the provision of healthcare to the provision of pastoral care *within* healthcare. New state run healthcare facilities were built alongside the investment of public funds in the development of existing healthcare facilities run by religious orders. Decreasing vocations to religious life in Ireland and the recognition of the specialised clinical and governance expertise necessary to run healthcare facilities also contributed to a changing landscape. The governance and regulation of formerly religiously run healthcare facilities has reflected these changes. Although some healthcare systems continue to be run with a strong religious ethos, nonetheless the overall governance has been devolved to lay experts. The context of this chapter is based in the Republic of Ireland where religious institutions (the vast majority run by the Catholic Church and a minority by the Church of Ireland and the Religious Society of Friends) provided much of the overall healthcare provision in the early years of the formation of the state in the early twentieth century. Hospitals recognised, valued and supported the appointment of chaplains by the churches and in most cases, chaplains were ordained or religious men and women and appointed by the local bishop or denomination. They were deemed qualified by virtue of their ordination/religious status.

In recent decades, there has been a growing appreciation of the importance of the education of healthcare chaplains, and this has been particularly the case since the introduction of CPE in Ireland in 1981. CPE has been the main methodology of education for healthcare ministry since then, and in recent years other programmes have evolved as well. The role of CPE and how it has shaped the educational landscape for healthcare chaplaincy and continues to evolve will be further explored in the second part of this chapter.

4 A Dual Relationship

The appointment of chaplains to healthcare institutions has hitherto been strongly influenced by local religious leaders – usually bishops – and in practice, healthcare chaplains in Ireland have (had) a dual relationship with their religious community and with the healthcare institution. This dual role or relationship has not been without tension, and it is recognised that chaplains can feel somewhat torn and not fully part of either community and feeling somewhat on the edge of both (Cobb 2013). In some ways, it could be described as a disenfranchised or dislocated space between being an insider and an outsider in both the healthcare institution and the church or religious community.

This raises a number of pertinent questions about the place of modern 'Christian healthcare chaplaincy'. Is the chaplain a representative of their faith/denomination in the healthcare institution, and thereby an extension of the faith community of the chaplain? Is there a distinction between religious care that is bound by the laws of a particular church and a broader approach to pastoral/spiritual care in a modern healthcare facility? Is the personal faith of the chaplain performative or formative? What are the expectations of the healthcare institution and the Christian community for Christian healthcare chaplains? What is the role of broader spiritual care, of which faith-specific care is one part? How do these questions relate with the recognition of the healthcare chaplain as a healthcare professional and spiritual care expert in an integrated interdisciplinary healthcare team? These questions have already presented themselves in other contexts similar to Ireland, such as the United Kingdom and in particular Scotland (MacLaren 2021; Nolan 2021).

As healthcare chaplaincy has evolved as an increasingly recognised profession within healthcare, this has also been supported by the growing recognition, research and value of the spiritual and religious dimensions of health and wellbeing. Indeed, the World Health Organization has grappled with the importance of the spiritual and religious dimensions of health and wellbeing since its founding in 1948 (Peng-Keller, Winiger, and Rauch 2022). The field of palliative care has made a particular contribution in this regard as the spiritual dimension of pain has been recognised alongside physical and psychological elements of suffering and worthy of attention (World Health Organization 2020). This has been enriched further by the development of the consensus definition of spirituality by Puchalski et al. in 2009 and developed further in 2013 as follows: 'Spirituality is a dynamic and intrinsic aspect of humanity through which persons seek ultimate meaning, purpose, and transcendence, and experience relationship to self, family, others, community, society, nature, and the significant or sacred. Spirituality is expressed through beliefs, values, traditions, and practices.' (Puchalski et al. 2014, 642–56). Of note in the development in this definition between 2009–2013 is the recognition of the expression of spirituality. We also know that spirituality is important to patients as they face illness and end-of-life and that attention to spiritual needs is integral to person centred healthcare (Clyne et al. 2019; Balboni et al. 2022).

5 An Evolving Relationship

Healthcare chaplains in Ireland (as is the case in many parts of the world), for the most part, require the nomination or endorsement of a faith community (usually a bishop or religious leader) to gain certification or accreditation as a healthcare chaplain and in turn to be eligible for appointment in the health service. It remains the case, however, that religious leaders can still nominate an ordained 'chaplain' without formal or recognised training or certification in healthcare chaplaincy. It is increasingly recognised however that this is not best practice and one that has caused concern amongst healthcare chaplains (including some of those appointed to these roles without adequate training) and other healthcare professionals. For some, this is an area of tension that undermines the professional recognition of the discipline, for others it is a convenient way to provide religious care to a particular cohort of patients. In the latter instance, this also raises the issue of the role of religious care, which in previous decades had a primacy in chaplaincy care. However, in an increasingly pluralist society, this approach requires attention and balance.

6 A Liminal Space

The dual relationship that chaplains can feel between the healthcare institution and their faith/belief community is in many ways a liminal space. This position as both insider and outsider is one that holds many opportunities for the chaplain to experience, embody and practice in a way that brings rich awareness of and to the often disconnected/ing experience of illness and frailty. It is in this space that the professionally trained chaplain can inhabit their role with confidence, safety and transformative skilled care in the overall spiritual care of patients and their loved ones. This liminal space provided the context for my care of Joy and her parents when they experienced distress, anguish, grief and uncertainty; questions that would not be answered meaningfully for them by a religious approach. This liminal space offered me the freedom to meet the individual needs of this unique family on their terms. My approach required me to discern and cherish their particular values and to provide expert spiritual care working closely with interdisciplinary colleagues in obstetrics, midwifery, social work and ultrasonography.

The spiritual care of Joy and her parents included an acknowledgement of their love, hopes and dreams, alongside holding the space for them to express their fears, loss and disappointment. In the provision of spiritual care, I adopted a narrative approach which supported Joy's parents as they recorded the story of their daughter through memory making, meaning making and building connections of love at each ultrasound scan (Nuzum 2018). It also involved the creation of a memory book where they wrote to Joy and shared their love and experiences throughout her short life in pregnancy and following her birth. As I responded to the spiritual needs of Joy's family, I did so from the confidence of my own beliefs and values as a Christian, without the need to impose my personal beliefs. As a professional Christian healthcare chaplain, this embodies the core competency to meet the client and to assist them in their values/belief system as they seek to make meaning and navigate their spiritual journey (ACPE-Ireland 2023; CAB 2014). It is an example of how the chaplain inhabits and engages in multiple spiritualities (Lasair 2020).

7 Increasing Religious Diversity

Ireland has experienced a marked change in religious/spiritual diversity in recent decades. In 1981, 93.1% of the population identified as Roman Catholic, in 2022 this was 69% (Central Statistics Office 2022). The number of those identifying as 'no religion' in 1981 was 1% and in 2022 was 14% (Central Statistics Office 2016). In response to this increasing diversity, healthcare chaplaincy has the opportunity to broaden far beyond the margins of religious identity yet still cherishing that identity for those for whom it is important – including for the chaplain. In my practice I meet many people who were formed in a Christian tradition but who no longer practice. When faced with illness, some return to the blueprint of their childhood formation to seek support, while others are repelled by it and react against a religious 'presentation' of spiritual care.

I also meet an increasing number of people who identity as 'spiritual but not religious' for whom the broadest sense of spirituality and meaning are essential support. In common with the broader European experience, religious and spiritual diversity in Ireland is continuously evolving, including within religious traditions and churches. In addition, there are many who 'believe (in something) without belonging (to any particular church)' (Davie 1990). For me, this is a fascinating and engaging context to be a healthcare chaplain – although I find more and more that the terms 'pastoral carer' or 'spiritual carer' are more accessible to those I care for. The word 'chaplain' for many carries a burden of religious weight, for others it is synonymous with spiritual care. The term chaplain is still the one formally used, although increasingly there is a shift in many places to the term 'pastoral care'. However, the formal salary code in our health service salary scale refers to 'Hospital Chaplain' – interestingly, it had previously been named 'Roman Catholic Hospital Chaplain'.

Notwithstanding the nomenclature, Christian healthcare chaplaincy is well-placed to embrace diversity as a gift. In this regard, the 'Christian' healthcare chaplain can and must remain authentic to their spiritual identity, while meaningfully and skilfully responding to the needs of those who do not share the particular Christian outlook of the chaplain, yet by virtue of being human will have spiritual needs, desires and expectations. This is akin to what MacLaren proposes as a 'third way' where the identity of the chaplain is the source of their professional identity (MacLaren 2021). It was from this place of my personal 'Christian' identity that I felt competent and authentic in meeting the spiritual needs of Joy's family in a meaningful way. They in turn knew that I was Christian and were comfortable receiving care that was sensitive to their values and, for my part, being a professional chaplain who does not impose my beliefs on others. For me, this spiritual 'breadth' is indeed the 'breath' for the inclusion and flourishing of Christian healthcare chaplaincy.

This leads to the place of the identity of the chaplain. Clinical Pastoral Education provides a robust and transformative education to develop and integrate the personal, pastoral and professional identity of the chaplain through the intensity of the CPE reflective and interpersonal process. So, what is the place of the identity of the Christian healthcare chaplain in an increasingly diverse and pluralist society? Some will question if there is a place for a 'Christian healthcare chaplain' beyond care with patients/service users who share the faith of the chaplain – and argue that, with a changing demography, there is a decreasing need. As a specialised spiritual carer, I argue that the Christian healthcare chaplain embodies their tradition and faith as a formative resource, rather than being a performer of it – something further expanded on in a number of chapters in this volume. The identity and spiritual formation of the Christian chaplain in this case is an essential element in the recognition of spiritual 'wisdom', integrity and maturity of the chaplain, and it is from this well-developed and integrated place that the Christian chaplain can minister to others. The integrity and authenticity of the chaplain will texture the spiritual care relationship with the patient/client. In my experience and research as a chaplain and chaplain educator, this evolving context opens exciting, creative, expansive, responsible, professionalised and rewarding opportunities for the contribution of Christian healthcare chaplains working in a pluralist and often complex healthcare environment alongside, and with, chaplains of other faiths and value systems. The Christian healthcare chaplain has much to offer.

8 The Distinctiveness of Chaplaincy

One of the challenges facing spiritual care and chaplaincy has been the challenge to articulate the distinctiveness of chaplaincy and spiritual care when it moves beyond purely religious parameters. The decrease in religious practice for some questions the need for healthcare chaplains – if religious care is their sole or primary *modus operandi*. This in part no doubt contributes to a sense of fear or loss for chaplains who practice primarily in religious ways. So how do chaplains articulate the particularity or value of what spiritual care is, or what healthcare chaplaincy offers to the healthcare environment for patients/clients, staff and for the institution as a whole?

Put simply, healthcare chaplains are the spiritual care experts in the interdisciplinary healthcare team. We are the experts in spirituality and spiritual issues that arise in the care of the human person. We are brokers of advocacy, dignity, meaning, adjustment and response to illness, trauma, and moral/existential challenge and complexity. You will discern a significant ethical expertise intertwined in this claim. Healthcare chaplains have the ability to 'be with' patients in an embodied, relational way that connects with their spiritual experience(s) of illness. This was my approach in my care of Joy and her young parents as they faced an uncertain future and realignment of hopes and dreams, love and loss. It is in this space that our identity as Christian healthcare chaplains serves us well to respond with spiritual generosity, spaciousness, authenticity and integrity. While the focus of this volume is Christian healthcare chaplaincy, the same can, of course, be said of any professional chaplain with a mature personal spiritual identity. These are core competencies that are developed incrementally and reflectively in a process such as CPE. The healthcare chaplain should be the reflective practitioner *par excellence* in the healthcare team. There are exciting opportunities for Christian chaplains to contribute meaningfully in a pluralist environment that is enriched with diversity of belief, values and approaches. In this way, faith values are included alongside broader spiritual and secular values that pertain to spirituality in healthcare.

Returning to Joy and her family, I would argue that it was the professional and skilled chaplain who was able to recognise and respond most meaningfully to the spiritual needs and furthermore to the co-creation of meaning making, appropriate expression or 'ritual' as her parents navigated the landscape of love, loss and memory making. Undoubtedly others in the team recognised the depth of distress and provided valuable and essential care, but the spiritual dimension was enhanced, and the overall care experience enriched with integrated spiritual care and the expression of what was an intensely spiritual experience. Although they had no particular faith tradition, Mary and Christophe came to terms with the impending death of Joy and sought to find meaning and value in her all too short physical life in which they sought to find spiritual meaning. For example, they described their sense of connection, of feeling her presence with them after she died.

9 The Conflict of Dual Relationships

How might the Christian healthcare chaplain have responded, had Joy's parents requested a termination of pregnancy, if that choice was in direct moral conflict with the views of the chaplain or the church they represent? Termination is now a legal option in Ireland following the diagnosis of a life-limiting condition in pregnancy that meets particular thresholds defined in the recently introduced Termination of Pregnancy legislation in 2018 (Government of Ireland 2018). This ethical challenge has become a new reality for maternity healthcare chaplains in Ireland. When faced with perinatal death, Christian maternity healthcare chaplains often navigate the space of inner conflict as they deal with perinatal death and the role of a loving God in the death of an infant (Nuzum et al. 2015; Nuzum, Meaney, and O'Donoghue 2016). I have had a number of conversations with chaplaincy colleagues about their experiences following the introduction of termination of pregnancy in 2019. One chaplain articulated "my role is to care with compassion and professionalism even if my church says it is wrong" and another "why should I be expected to care for people who choose to end a baby's life?". In these two statements there is the reality of the tensions of dual accountability. It is not the place of this chapter to adjudicate, but rather to open up the question about how chaplains navigate this morally and ethically challenging space. Ethically, the primacy of the care of patients should be uppermost (Laoire et al. 2021). For me, I find a congruence between being able to meaningfully provide spiritual care for someone whose views I do not share and also being able to care for someone who has to make a very difficult decision about the life of their child even if I would not have made that decision for myself. This requires a high level of self-awareness, spiritual maturity and the openness to explore these inner conflicts in supervision.

10 CPE and Healthcare Chaplaincy Education

Modern healthcare requires all healthcare professionals to commit to the highest standards of evidence-based practice, education and research. It goes without saying that the same should apply to healthcare chaplains. The evidence base for healthcare chaplaincy has grown significantly in recent years and is well illustrated in this volume. The preparation and education of Christian healthcare chaplains require action and commitment both on the spiritual, theological and personal formation of the chaplain as a person of faith, and a commitment to robust integrative education to be a competent and effective spiritual care expert and practitioner: a professional amongst professionals. In common with other professional disciplines, the ongoing education, professional development and specialisation of healthcare chaplains is crucial. This will demonstrate that healthcare chaplaincy is indeed a specialist spiritual care with considerable contribution to make to the healing, recovery, wellbeing and experience of patients in healthcare alongside an increasingly recognised role in the 'community' of the healthcare institution and staff support/wellbeing.

CPE had its beginnings in the development of the chaplain in a clinical context. As a transformative educational process, CPE has been challenged to adapt and align more with developments in the scholarship of teaching and learning (SoTL) and broader healthcare educational developments. In recent years, the provision of CPE in Ireland has been following these approaches with the introduction of competency-based assessment and the development of a number of international reciprocal arrangements between the Association of Clinical Pastoral Education (Ireland) Ltd with CPE education in Canada, the USA and New Zealand. CPE in Ireland has been following the pattern of 'units' each with four hundred hours balanced between clinical experience and didactic/group/interpersonal work and reflection. It is provided at two incremental levels (Level 1 and level 2) for healthcare chaplains/spiritual care professionals in accordance with nationally agreed standards. The developments in CPE education in Ireland continue to evolve to prepare chaplains/pastoral carers to be professional healthcare chaplains in modern healthcare. An important shift in recent years has been to have a greater appreciation for the gifts, wisdom and experience of CPE participants as adult learners and the importance of the development of core skills in the provision of spiritual care to all. I experience this as a recognition of a 'relational pedagogy' between educator and CPE participant in the creative and robust learning and growth (Bovill 2020).[1] In addition, the methodology of CPE and some of the content from CPE programmes has been used to provide academically accredited generalist spiritual care programmes at university level for other healthcare professionals. CPE centres have also been providing continuing professional development opportunities for healthcare chaplains and other healthcare professionals. Further work is needed to bring CPE more fully into academic structures in Ireland to facilitate inclusion in and recognition of CPE at an academic level.

1 See the chapter of Trace Haythorn, this volume.

11 CPE and Healthcare: A Natural Synergy

The growing recognition of the importance of compassion and dignity in person-centred healthcare by the wider healthcare world, coupled with a shift from a former paternalistic approach to a client-centred partnership in health and healthcare, has opened opportunities for healthcare chaplaincy and CPE to play a particular role. A seminal paper in *The Lancet* on the need for a transformed medical curriculum identified three dimensions of learning that are apposite in the healthcare community: informative, formative and transformative (Frenk et al. 2010). These insights place the CPE approach well in the overall congruence of the educational approach for healthcare professionals. Moreover, the growing awareness in recent years of the need to move from a paternalistic to a person-centred model of education and care is well aligned with the didactic approach of CPE as the personal, pastoral and professional identity of the healthcare chaplain is developed in a relational way for healthcare chaplaincy ministry (Jones 2010; Vanderstelt, Van Dijk, and Lasair 2023; 2023; Hilsman 2018; Doherty and Nuzum 2023).

There is a natural synergy between this appreciation and the approach of CPE in the development of the person as a professional and their ability to relate at a human level in healthcare. As evidenced above, the skills and approach of CPE are eminently transferable to other areas of healthcare. Anecdotally, it was feedback from other healthcare professionals to our CPE students that prompted the provision of an adapted form of CPE for healthcare professionals that has been running successfully in our hospital and university since 2016 (CPD 2018). This programme has been consistently highly evaluated by healthcare professionals from general practice, medicine, midwifery, physiotherapy, psychotherapy and social care. This initiative is mirrored by similar novel programmes of interprofessional spiritual care education in other countries and seeks to develop the generalist approach to spiritual care while at the same time supporting the specialist nature and training of CPE for healthcare chaplains.

There are exciting opportunities for CPE to continue this academic and wider healthcare integration while maintaining a firm commitment to the distinctiveness of personal, pastoral and professional growth of the healthcare chaplain, and an appreciation of core spiritual care qualities – such as presence, empathy, vulnerability etc. that are perhaps not measurable in a traditional sense. Yet, these are qualities that are increasingly recognized as key in all healthcare relationships. In an increasingly specialized medical world, where disease and illness are understood and investigated with extraordinary precision, spiritual care brings a valuable contribution to seeing the human person as a whole. To remember the person in their wholeness with exquisite empathy, pastoral skill, professional pastoral intervention and transformative presence. For some, this will be met by a religious response, for others it will require a generic one, and for all a mature and skilled spiritual skill set, breadth, and rootedness on the part of the chaplain.

To return finally to Joy. Joy lived for three hours following her birth. Following advanced planning, her parents Mary and Christophe were able to value every moment of her short life. I was honoured to be asked to meet Joy and with her parents, we gave her her name in a ritual of love as her mum held her close to her breast and embraced by her dad. Joy's parents have treasured memories, photographs and video footage. As their spiritual carer, I joined them for a short while to celebrate these important moments and, importantly, also withdrew to the background so that their finite family time was theirs. A few days following her death, I accompanied Christophe and Mary as they invited close family members to say goodbye to Joy, and much of the story we had created together was used to shape the farewell ritual. Mary and Christophe were in touch with me over the coming year as they reflected on their experience and their continuing bonds of love with their daughter Joy. They experienced and appreciated the openness of spiritual hospitality in their liminal space of grief and loss in pregnancy and birth as they grew to cherish, love, hold, greet, parent, bid farewell to and now to remember with profound tenderness, Joy who will always be their daughter and continues to have an active place in their family. As a chaplain, I was inspired by and sought to embody the breadth and breath of spiritual care.

References

ACPE-Ireland. 2023. 'ACPE-Ireland'. 2023. www.acpeireland.com.

Balboni, Tracy A, Tyler J Van der Weele, Stephanie D Doan-Soares, Katelyn NG Long, Betty R Ferrell, George Fitchett, Harold G Koenig, Paul A Bain, Christina Puchalski, and Karen E Steinhauser. 2022. 'Spirituality in Serious Illness and Health'. Journal of the American Medical Association 328 (2): 184–97.

Bovill, Catherine. 2020. Co-Creating Learning and Teaching: Towards Relational Pedagogy in Higher Education. Critical Practice in Higher Education. St Albans: Critical Publishing Ltd.

CAB. 2014. 'Certification of Healthcare Chaplains and Recognised Standards'. Chaplaincy Accreditation Board, House of Bishops of the Church of Ireland. http://ireland.anglican.org/cmsfiles/pdf/Information/Resources/hob/2014.003.pdf.

Central Statistics Office. 2016. 'Census of Population 2016 – Profile 8 Irish Travellers, Ethnicity and Religion'. Central Statistics Office.

Central Statistics Office. 2022. 'Census of Population 2022 -Migration and Diversity'. Central Statistics Office.

Clyne, Barbara, Sinead M O'Neill, Daniel Nuzum, Michelle O'Neill, James Larkin, Máirín Ryan, and Susan M Smith. 2019. 'Patients' Spirituality Perspectives at the End of Life: A Qualitative

Evidence Synthesis'. BMJ Supportive & Palliative Care. https://doi.org/10.1136/bmjspcare-2019-002016.
Cobb, Mark. 2013. 'The Location and Identity of Chaplains: A Contextual Model'. Health and Social Care Chaplaincy, April, 10–15. https://doi.org/10.1558/hscc.v7i2.10.
CPD. 2018. 'An Introduction to Clinical Pastoral Education for Healthcare Professionals'. University College Cork. 2018. https://www.ucc.ie/en/cpd/options/medhealth/cpd1621/.
Davie, Grace. 1990. 'Believing without Belonging: Is This the Future of Religion in Britain?' Social Compass 37 (4): 455–69. https://doi.org/10.1177/003776890037004004.
Doherty, John Patrick, and Daniel Nuzum. 2023. '"Can You See What I Say?" Beyond Words: Pastoral Care Education and Practice Among the Deaf and Hard of Hearing Community'. Health and Social Care Chaplaincy 11 (2): 205–19. https://doi.org/10.1558/hscc.25862.
Frenk, Julio, Lincoln Chen, Zulfiqar A Bhutta, Jordan Cohen, Nigel Crisp, Timothy Evans, Harvey Fineberg, et al. 2010. 'Health Professionals for a New Century: Transforming Education to Strengthen Health Systems in an Interdependent World'. The Lancet 376 (9756): 1923–58. https://doi.org/10.1016/S0140-6736(10)61854-5.
Government of Ireland. 2018. Health (Regulation of Termination of Pregnancy) Act 2018. 31. https://www.irishstatutebook.ie/eli/2018/act/31/enacted/en/pdf.
Hilsman, Gordon J. 2018. How to Get the Most Out of Clinical Pastoral Education. 1st ed. London ; Philadelphia: Jessica Kingsley Publishers.
Jones, Logan C. 2010. 'You Learn It in Your Heart: Transformative Learning Theory and Clinical Pastoral Education'. Journal of Pastoral Care & Counseling: Advancing Theory and Professional Practice through Scholarly and Reflective Publications 64 (4): 1–10. https://doi.org/10.1177/154230501006400407.
Laoire, Áine Ni, Daniel Nuzum, Maeve O'Reilly, Marie Twomey, Keelin O'Donoghue, and Mary Devins. 2021. 'Perinatal Palliative Care'. In Oxford Textbook of Palliative Care for Children, edited by Richard Hain, Ann Goldman, Adam Rapoport, Michelle Meiring, Richard Hain, Ann Goldman, Adam Rapoport, and Michelle Meiring, 3rd ed., 325–31. Oxford, UK: Oxford University Press. https://doi.org/10.1093/med/9780198821311.003.0029.
Lasair, Simon. 2020. 'What's the Point of Clinical Pastoral Education and Pastoral Counselling Education? Political, Developmental, and Professional Considerations'. Journal of Pastoral Care & Counseling: Advancing Theory and Professional Practice through Scholarly and Reflective Publications 74 (1): 22–32. https://doi.org/10.1177/1542305019897563.
MacLaren, Duncan. 2021. 'All Things to All People? The Integrity of Spiritual Care in a Plural Health Service'. Health and Social Care Chaplaincy 9 (1): 27–41. https://doi.org/10.1558/hscc.40568.
Nolan, Steve. 2021. 'Religious, Spiritual, Pastoral . . . and Secular? Where Next for Chaplaincy?' Health and Social Care Chaplaincy 9 (1): 1–10. https://doi.org/10.1558/hscc.42735.
Nuzum, Daniel. 2018. 'Giving Voice to the Story. Working with Patients Who Cannot Speak'. In Paediatric Chaplaincy: Principles, Practices and Skills, edited by Paul Nash, Mark Bartel, and Sally Nash, 167–76. London, UK: Jessica Kinglsey Publishers.
Nuzum, Daniel, Sarah Meaney, and Keelin O'Donoghue. 2016. 'The Provision of Spiritual and Pastoral Care Following Stillbirth in Ireland: A Mixed Methods Study'. BMJ Supportive & Palliative Care 6 (2): 194–200. https://doi.org/10.1136/bmjspcare-2013-000533.
Nuzum, Daniel, Sarah Meaney, Keelin O'Donoghue, and Heather Morris. 2015. 'The Spiritual and Theological Issues Raised by Stillbirth for Healthcare Chaplains'. Journal of Pastoral Care & Counseling: Advancing Theory and Professional Practice through Scholarly and Reflective Publications 69 (3): 163–70. https://doi.org/10.1177/1542305015602714.

Peng-Keller, Simon, Fabian Winiger, and Raphael Rauch. 2022. The Spirit of Global Health: The World Health Organization and the 'Spiritual Dimension' of Health, 1946–2021. Oxford, New York: Oxford University Press.

Puchalski, Christina M, Robert Vitillo, Sharon K Hull, and Nancy Reller. 2014. 'Improving the Spiritual Dimension of Whole Person Care: Reaching National and International Consensus'. Journal of Palliative Medicine 17 (6): 642–56. https://doi.org/10.1089/jpm.2014.9427.

Vanderstelt, Heather, Alida Van Dijk, and Simon Lasair. 2023. 'Transformational Education: Exploring the Lasting Impact of Students' Clinical Pastoral Education Experiences'. Journal of Health Care Chaplaincy 29 (1): 89–104. https://doi.org/10.1080/08854726.2022.2040892.

World Health Organization. 2020. 'Palliative Care'. World Health Organization. 5 August 2020. https://www.who.int/news-room/fact-sheets/detail/palliative-care.

Traugott Roser

From Pastoral Care to Specialized Spiritual Care. Envisioning Future Models from Personal Experience in the Past

Abstract: Pastoral care – in its essence – is a meaningful encounter between two or more people sharing experience, burdens and needs, emotions, and resources of faith, hope, and love in a situation of vulnerability. What makes these encounters Christian is the possibility that Christ's presence can be recognised in hindsight, by reflecting on them through Scripture. The article reflects on the author's personal pathways as healthcare chaplain and as receiver of spiritual care, and theoretically framed models for future specialized spiritual care as part of a multiprofessional team. It covers aspects of training in the tradition of CPE, the importance of academic theological education, interdisciplinary research, and the moral dimension of spiritual care. One part of being a chaplain is artful use of skills and technique; the other part is personal experience based in both individual spiritual life and lived Christian faith. Christian healthcare chaplains belong to two living bodies, linking the body of Christ and the functional organism that is the healthcare system.

1 Linking Two Bodies – The Dual Role of Healthcare Chaplains

The 'tension' Christian healthcare chaplains experience in their dual performance as representatives of a specific faith community and as part of a multi-professional healthcare team has sometimes been described as challenging, demanding, or even alienating. Some serve as ordained ministers, some as theologically trained lay professionals. In many Western countries Christian chaplains often represent a denomination that once was dominant in their country or region (Roman Catholic in Belgium, parts of the Netherlands, Switzerland, Germany, Church of England, Lutheran/Reformed in Scandinavian countries and parts of Germany and Switzerland) but has seen dwindling influence in a growingly secular public space. To identify oneself as representative of a specific faith tradition, thus, needs ongoing and critical reflection on one's church history, theological formation, and call to professional ministry. Some of the papers in this volume document an awareness for the challenges, and sometimes obstacles and scepticism faith communities must

https://doi.org/10.1515/9783112205839-009

face. Healthcare chaplains, however, serve with a diaconal mission to care for and be with persons affected by illness (patients, family and friends, staff) within secular settings not dominated by religious orders or faith traditions, but by evidence-based medicine, and restrictive financial budgets. Thus, dual belonging comes with a sense of equidistance towards both faith community and the health system.

Chaplains' academic training, religious language, use of symbols and modes of action sets them apart from other healthcare professionals, resulting in a sense of 'otherness'. Working within the medical and hierarchical setting of healthcare institutions and being constantly confronted with physical and psychological illness, curing, healing, dying, and recovering, can also set healthcare chaplains apart from parish life and ministry. However, as I want to explore more deeply in the following, this tension can be understood as a resource. The opportunity of equally belonging to two different social systems can be understood in a metaphorical way reminiscent of Pauline semantics: Christians, through baptism and by ways of the call of the Spirit, belong to one body (cf. 1 Corinthians 12:13), in fact, they are the body of Christ (cf. Galatians 3:28). Furthermore, as healthcare professionals, chaplains are also members of an – at best – organically functioning body focusing on one goal shared by all: curing and caring for, healing and treating ill persons. In all otherness, dual belonging can bring out the best in Christian chaplaincy as a genuine contribution of the Christian call to healing under the conditions of today's healthcare system(s) and within pluralistic societies. Chaplains link two bodies, being rooted and having one foot in two fields each.

The following reflections follow a path between the author's personal experience as a healthcare chaplain and theological reasoning. Personal experience in the field of healthcare is a continuous, embodied process of learning and understanding. This approach follows the road taken by the fathers and mothers of Christian pastoral care and of the hospice movement. Their teaching, research, and conceptualizing the art of pastoral (Anton T Boisen, see Boisen 1971) and palliative care (Cicely Saunders, see Saunders and Clark 2006) is deeply rooted in personal experience, Christian faith tradition, and academic work.

1.1 Pastoral Care and Clinical Bioethics

Personal experience: For a couple of years, the Lutheran Church in Bavaria assigned me the role of coordinator of medical-ethical questions. The job was to provide church leaders with expert knowledge in case they were asked about the church's position in public discourse. The main issues in the early 2000s were advance directives, perinatal death, late-term abortion, autonomy of persons with dementia, and organ transplantation. By inviting practitioners from medical professions and clinical pastoral care, patient advocates and ethicists to participate in round table discussions, it was possible to develop guidelines for practical use within the clinical context and for parish pastors, but also for synods responsible for official public statements. Organizing round table talks, I was introduced to the complex reality healthcare chaplains had to face in the field of clinical bioethics. Counselling, pastoral care, and the performance of liturgies take place in critical conflict situations. While there was not much chaplaincy-specific literature on these issues in Germany, the Center for Clinical Bioethics at the Kennedy Institute of Ethics at Georgetown University in Washington D.C., USA, offered plenty of resources from Northern America, Great Britain, and Australia. Oftentimes, however, this was provided by authors and researchers in the field of philosophy (like Edmund Pellegrino, see Bulger and McGovern 2001), or by health professionals (like Carol Taylor, see Taylor and Dell'Oro 2006).

Chaplains are able to link different systems and to mediate – in questions of clinical bioethics – between their faith community, specialized health professionals, affected persons, and academic theology.

Within the last ten to fifteen years, research provided insights into the involvement of healthcare chaplains in ethical counselling, decision-making, and teaching. In Germany, Thorsten Moos and colleagues published findings of a theological study among healthcare chaplains (Moos et al. 2016). Stefanie Clemm published a pilot survey on the role of 141 Christian healthcare chaplains in end-of-life decision-making in Germany as part of a multi-professional research team that combined physicians, ethicists, palliative care specialists and chaplains. Participating chaplains reported being confronted with decisions concerning the limitations of life-sustaining treatment on average two to three times per month (Clemm et al. 2015). The pilot study was able to show that integration of chaplains within multi-professional teams was connected to a significantly higher satisfaction rate with ethical decisions made and with the communication process. Pastoral caregivers reported a "dual role" as both representatives of their faith community and specialized healthcare professional.

It was, however, surprising that only a small minority (only 7%) of healthcare chaplains considered themselves as representing their church and their church's teaching on ethical questions, while most of them define themselves as their patients' advocate (67%) or as a facilitator of communication processes (61%) (cf. Clemm et al. 2015, 49). It did not make much of a difference whether chaplains were well integrated within multi-professional teams or part of the administrative body: representing the church, its teachings, and positions in moral decision making does not seem to be a role healthcare chaplains like to accept for themselves.

Nevertheless, the dual role of Christian chaplains as connected to their faith community on the one hand, and on the other hand, as spiritual care professionals integrated in a multi-professional healthcare setting, emerged as a theme that needed further research.

Building on these findings and on Lindsay B. Carey's (2012) and others' research, Sebastian Farr and colleagues conducted a quantitative survey among German-speaking healthcare chaplains in Austria, Germany, and Switzerland (Farr, Roser, and Coors 2023). One-hundred and fifty-four, mostly protestant chaplains participated, with three quarters of them (75.3%) funded by their church, 11.4% (n=18) by the hospital they worked in, the rest by other sponsors. The study was most interested in specific fields of ethical conflicts in the praxis of healthcare chaplains. Supporting findings of Carey (2012), the survey found an emphasis on questions surrounding the end of life. Contact with end of life-questions happens often during direct pastoral care visits or by referral through nursing staff. Interprofessional cooperation seems to lead to a concept of spiritual care centred on coordinating the spiritual care practice of healthcare professionals with that of specialized spiritual care, a distinction described by Peng-Keller (Peng-Keller 2020).

Not known, however, is how pastoral care counselling on ethical issues relates to faith-community-specific praxis, i.e., confession, prayer, ritual, and pastoral conversation. Or, to put it differently: are ethical counselling, moral orientation, and normative, religious communication related, and if so, how? If there is a connection between faith-based pastoral care and clinical ethics counselling, both are linked in the *gestalt* of one professional person and his or her *habitus* (cf. Bourdieu 2023): the chaplain. This applies to both structured forms of ethics deliberation where chaplains present themselves as religious actors, and to nonstructured forms of communication or unplanned pastoral care visits where chaplains function as experts of open communication and trust-based relations.

Fields of interest in this regard are a) questions of perinatal death including faith-related ritual and sacramental forms of pastoral care to stillborn infants (e.g. baptismal services) and in the case of late-stage abortion after prenatal diagnostics (e.g. interfaith funeral services), and b) questions of pastoral care and counselling in the context of hastened death, death wish, physician assisted suicide, and euthanasia. What does it mean to conceptualize and experience a faith-community based pastor as "hopeful presence" (Nolan 2011) in morally ambivalent situations within healthcare institutions that are not in line with normative church teachings? There is a potential tension resulting from the dual belonging of healthcare chaplains. It can, however, also be described as an openness to link the offerings of the traditions of faith communities with crisis and conflict situations within the clinical setting. The basic question is whether there is a distinction between an open spiritual care concept that conceptualizes specific spiritual care according to qualification and professional training, and faith community-related pastoral care in terms of "handling" and managing normative conflicts.

1.2 Being a Member of a Multi-Professional Healthcare Team Opens New Horizons

In 2004, my church assigned me to a new project to pastoral care in palliative care at a large university hospital, as the Protestant part of a joint ecumenical venture with the Roman Catholic Archdiocese of Munich and Freising. The university had just recently established a clinical centre for Palliative Medicine that was supposed to integrate chaplaincy as part of whole person care. Both assigned chaplains, one Roman-Catholic, the other Lutheran, were asked to absolve CPE-training for the new job. While being members of the hospital's ecumenical pastoral care department, my Roman Catholic colleague and I were also members of the multiprofessional palliative care team. Being a member of the palliative care team meant bedside care and counselling with patients and family members, participating in rounds and ethics committee meetings, team-supervision, providing pastoral care to staff members, and teaching assignments in spiritual and palliative care to medical students, and palliative care training programs. While the project was based in palliative care, it raised questions considering the inclusion of spiritual care issues familiar to palliative medicine and hospice care into the wider fields of healthcare chaplaincy and more traditional pastoral care. Research projects like, among others, the development of a German version of the FICA tool (Borneman, Ferrell, and Puchalski 2010) and taking a spiritual history (Paal et al. 2017) reach beyond palliative care and benefit from an interdisciplinary research group with professionals from social work, psychotherapy, medicine, and nursing.

While seemingly well established in other countries, the term "spiritual care" raised many concerns among Christian healthcare chaplains in German-speaking countries as it was and still is associated with an unspecific concept of non-religious spirituality (Karle 2010; EKD 2023, 23–25) and the provision of generic spiritual care by other than faith-based professions (Nauer 2010), a trend described for the Netherlands by Wim Smeets in this volume. Concerns were also raised within the hospice-oriented spectrum of the field, when Birgit and Andreas Heller proposed a multireligious concept of spiritual care sceptical towards a Christian and church-promoted claim to spiritual care as based in Christian tradition (Heller 2014). My experience, however, was quite different: Patients within a hospital usually come from diverse cultural backgrounds and different religious, non-religious and philosophical traditions. This was also the case on my ward. But once I would introduce myself as a Protestant pastor, patients would name their belonging and openly signal whether they would like to receive pastoral and spiritual care or not. More than in any other pastoral field I had experienced before, I met and worked with people from various traditions.

Working within the hospital, a highly professional surrounding and among intellectually intriguing specialists, and caring in vulnerable situations for patients, family members, and staff members of various backgrounds, I found my personal beliefs, spirituality, and existence affected, both challenging and making me grow. When my husband was diagnosed with incurable cancer, he was hospitalized, treated and taken care of at "my hospital". I learned to appreciate the team effort of the cancer care unit to provide whole person care until death. The twofold experience of being both provider and receiver of spiritual care was profoundly important in understanding what it means to be ill or suffering, how much help I/we would accept – and whom I/we would want as my/our spiritual care provider. I learned from the margins of my own fragmented existence (Luther 1991).

Again, on a more abstract level, my personal experience is rather symptomatic of the transformation of the provision from traditional Christian pastoral care towards spiritual care within healthcare institutions in German-speaking countries. Describing the duality of the chaplain's role of "representative of a (specific) faith community" and "specialized health professional" tends to individualize it as a challenge to the professional subject who has to personally deal with the demands of two different systems: the healthcare institution one works *in*, and the Christian faith community one works *for*. John Swinton (this volume) describes this in a similar way, but the other way around: "Christian theology and embodied Christian spirituality can enable the chaplain *at an individual level to negotiate* the complexities of working with people of all faiths and none" (cf. Swinton, this volume).

Rather than individualizing the problem, it could be better described in ways regarding two different systems in transition (Swinton calls it 'institutional spirituality'): the medical system that – starting in palliative and hospice care – has begun to include spiritual care as part of a holistic approach to healthcare. Since healthcare institutions are a part of a secular system, offering care to patients and family without regard to their religious or ideological affiliation, the inclusion of spiritual care needs to be on a fundamental level, open to different religious and non-religious traditions. However, the religious system that, to this day, provides professional pastoral care and training, is in a transitional process: on the one hand serving to an ever more diversified field of healthcare, on the other hand, with a dwindling amount of human resources.

Chris Swift (this volume) describes a similar process in England: the context of healthcare chaplaincy has "dramatically changed" during the last century, from a position of total control by the Church of England to a far more diversified field. In Germany, both leading Christian confessional church bodies (Roman Catholic and the different Protestant denominations) have reacted to the changing demand and the emergence of spiritual care by putting Christian pastoral care in constructive, yet critical relation to spiritual care (Sekretariat der Deutschen Bischofskonferenz 2022; EKD 2020). Practical theologian Günter Emlein refers to sociological system theory to describe chaplaincy as "hybride Praxis" (Emlein 2017, 86), constantly switching between either a religious code or a therapeutical code.[1]

The dual belonging of professional healthcare chaplains to both the religious system and a multiprofessional healthcare team, thus, is an ongoing process of linking two systems and transforming the medical place into a spiritually meaningful space: by ministering from a specific faith community and being theologically trained, chaplains bring a specific 'otherness' to the medically and therapeutically defined place. Following Martina Löw's sociology of space (Löw 2015) and Michel Foucault's concepts of heterotopy and heterochrony (Foucault 2013), the presence and the actions of Christian chaplains transform defined places into spaces of transcendence and spirituality. The presence of faith community-related healthcare chaplains in an otherwise medical setting enables the patient, family member, and members of the healthcare staff to deal with existential and personal issues raised by the constant confrontation with life, death, and crisis in a way that transcends the medical space.

As a consequence, healthcare chaplains need to be a) religious agents firmly based within a specific faith tradition, b) academically trained and hermeneutically competent theologians, c) well accustomed to the hospital setting, its language and customs, d) open to provide spiritual care to persons with spiritual backgrounds other than their own, and e) self-aware of their own vulnerability and needs. These aspects are the main issues of the White Paper on Christian Healthcare Chaplaincy, especially regarding core competencies and demands for education and training (Peng-Keller et al. 2025).

1 Wendy Cadge uses the term "code-switching", cf. Cadge and Sigalow (2013).

2 Singing Christmas Carols As Holistic Medical Goal: The Case of Mr. Smith

Belonging to the healthcare team, chaplains need to be transparent in their contribution to the goals of the multi-professional team. Are they a functioning member of the therapeutic body, contributing to palliative, curative, and rehabilitative support for patients, or are they dysfunctional?

Mr. Smith was 70 years old, married, with three adult children, a daughter and two sons. He belonged to a Protestant church. His wife and children had taken care of him over the past four years at home: he suffered from hypoxic brain injury, incurred during reanimation after a heart attack. During the last months he suffered from recurring pneumonia and a worsening general condition. After Mr. Smith was admitted to the ward, the team encountered him in a degenerative state during his first night. He was shaking, in a cold sweat and extremely cramped. When asked if he was in pain, or where he felt pain, he would repeat the last word spoken, saying «pain, pain, pain». It was difficult to understand whether this was his way of talking about his situation, or if it was an automated response (echolalia).

Prior to admission, Mr. Smith had stopped eating and drinking as his general condition had deteriorated to such a level that he and his family had accepted his pre-final situation. His family and his family physician agreed that ending food intake was Mr. Smith's deliberate decision to end his life. Throughout the next few days, his condition improved a little, which often occurs and is tellingly called the "Lazarus phenomenon". He enjoyed the nurse's care and started to hope that his overall condition could change for the better after years of deterioration.

When he partially got better and was even able to shower in the morning, sit in a lounge chair, begin to eat and drink again, he could sometimes give clear answers, and if he could not speak, would "smile the sweetest smile possible" (as the nurse put it). Everybody was confused about his will and intentions. It was Christmas and his family was in euphoria about this turn of events and changed their plans and began thinking of new forms of therapies for Mr. Smith. Finally, his twin sister came from abroad to stay with him and the rest of the family. On Christmas Eve, Mr. Smith sang Christmas carols with them.

This state of well-being did not last long, and he recessed into the condition in which he had arrived, unable to eat or drink anymore, and pneumonia returned. The reason for this change was unclear, leaving his caregivers in a situation of disorientation. No one in his family would give up hope that the high he had experienced would return.

Discussions of discontinuing life-prolonging therapies came up again. However, the patient's daughter was not able to follow along with this idea, unlike the rest of the family. The family, except for the daughter, denied the placement of a feeding tube according to his oral advance directive. The medical situation of the patient got worse rapidly until he, suddenly, became very pale and developed dyspnoea and lost consciousness. He died three days later on the ward. Finally, Mr. Smith himself had made a decision – despite all round table discussions and medical decisions – and had chosen his own way of ending his life.

As a chaplain, in the beginning I had not much of an idea about Mr. Smith's spirituality or faith. Spending silent hours at the bedside and in conversation with family members, I was able to get an idea, making use of consensus definitions of spirituality by Puchalski et al (2014) and Nolan et al. (2011).

Mr. Smith was firmly connected to his family, including his twin sister. They cared for him, respected his decisions and had taken care of him for a long time. They provided him with biographic information. Thus, the family took care of his connection to himself and things that were important to his identity. Part of this was that Mr. Smith was also connected to a specific faith tradition. Second, Mr. Smith expressed and experienced spirituality: He was able to celebrate Christmas together with his family and – singing Christmas carols – actively participated in this special time of the year, a deep faith experience on a deep level. Thirdly, Mr. Smith enjoyed being cared for, being caressed and touched in a sensitive and meaningful way. The improvement of his physical condition shows that the prime goal of palliative care was obviously reached: improvement of quality of life at the end of life. Shortly before death ending his life, Mr. Smith experienced the Kairos of a good life.

The spirituality of the family can be seen as a dynamic process dealing with a constantly changing existential situation. Acting in a situation of ambivalence, they sticked to the patient's will, working their way through issues of guilt and shame, freedom and responsibility, hope and despair, love and joy. Their loving connectedness to Mr. Smith (husband, father, brother) was challenged to its core by the question whether to continue nutrition or not. Nevertheless, they were able to connect with the patient, express their grief and sense of loss, and celebrate the time that they had together. In this situation, the chaplain's job was to offer time, presence, opportunity to clear their mind, and to confide things otherwise not openly uttered, and ritual, easing the pressure of medical decision-making.

Finally, in the case of caring for Mr. Smith, spiritual issues of the team were considered along with value-issues and the spiritual and religious foundations of one's own professional doing. Palliative care is a moral endeavour, as it aims to enable the patient and the family to experience quality of life up to the last minute. They follow an ideal of the good life in the face of finitude. The ups and downs of Mr. Smith's condition between curing and caring come into the way. However, the team felt they fulfilled the goal of hospice care to give life to the days and not days to life. Spiritual care in this situation is able to offer space to verbalize ambivalent feelings, either in an individual counselling setting, or within a team meeting. A chaplain is able to point at difficulties that some team members may have with therapeutic decisions, and to insist on forms of communication like round-table-discussions, team supervision, etc.

Coming from a palliative care background, the issue of healing is more than a curative understanding. Since spirituality in palliative care is a multifaceted and multilayered concept that regards not only the spirituality/religiosity of the patient, but also family members, and healthcare staff, healing and well-being have to be considered within a social frame as well as a physical, psychological, and spiritual frame. Chaplains contribute to a Christian understanding of healing that is neither restricted to the restitution of health as it was before the crisis, nor does it exclude this restoration. Healing has to be considered in a broader sense, including relational aspects which are an essential part of spirituality: the relation to oneself, to others, to God.

Simon Peng-Keller draws on biblical narratives to describe the healing processes told in the Gospel stories. They are not restricted to the restitution of physical or mental health. In their encounters with Jesus, persons in need of healing experience more than they sought for: a fullness of meaning transcending everything they perceived as meaningful. Looking back, they realize what kept them blind and excluded them from life (cf. Peng-Keller 2023). The question regarding the Christian call to health and healing, thus, raises the issue of healing effects of chaplaincy care.

In her doctoral thesis, Nika Höfler takes a Grounded Theory approach to a theologically sound understanding of the effectiveness of healthcare chaplaincy interventions (Höfler 2022). Analysing self-reported case narratives by professional chaplains and semi-structured interviews with patients and family members, "vulnerability" emerged as the core category with different dimensions: While the patient is in a state of being vulnerable in physical and psychological ways, his or her relations and social status are vulnerable, as well. Illness can be experienced as a spiritual crisis. This also applies to family members and health care staff members, leaving individuals and groups vulnerable. It is within these situations that healthcare chaplaincy gets involved.

2.1 Context

Chaplains are called in acute situations of heightened vulnerability in the physical and psychological dimensions of the patient. Chaplains are also called in situations of deficient communication between healthcare staff and patients that endanger the success of therapeutic measures or aspects of compliance or can be disruptive to the functioning of a complete ward. Pastoral ministry is 'on call' 24/7, and most often called in situations of crisis that can happen when other psychosocial staff members are off-duty. Traditionally, pastors could be called in order to provide rituals or 'last rites'; the custom of availability in situations of acute need has not changed, even as the demand for sacramental rites may have become less. Chaplains start communication, restore trust, facilitate case discussions, helping staff and family members to adapt to the situation. Healing, thus, means healing of context and relations.

2.2 Otherness

Chaplains act as representatives of religious teachings, faith-based institutions and traditions, and at the same time expose themselves as authentic persons with personal spirituality and beliefs. They themselves are vulnerable in and because of their role, often met with trust and scepticism in equal measure. Pastors' social position as healthcare chaplains is institutionally vulnerable: the fact that they are called upon in situations of institutional uncertainty and situations of dealing with death and dying, involves healthcare chaplains as specialists for managing contingency. The hospital is a place where staff members as well as chaplains are constantly confronted with existential situations and failure of therapeutic strategies. While many regard it as part of professional behaviour to be able to cope with these experiences, more often than not, existential pain can be infective (Gabl 2022). Chaplains, like other health professionals, are exposed to existential pain. Höfler found that chaplains very often describe themselves as being deeply affected by the situations they witness, both emotionally and theologically. As resonating entities, chaplains constantly re-adapt their theological perception to new experiences of the vulnerability of others and return to their own spiritual resources. Adaptation can be described as an ongoing hermeneutical process singular to chaplaincy both in healthcare and in other institutions such as the military, in trauma counselling, in correctional institutions, etc. One effect of chaplaincy that should not be neglected is the constant reconstructing of theological reasoning and religious performance, leading to the next subcategory of vulnerability.

To Christian healthcare chaplains, biblical texts, especially psalms of the Hebrew Bible and Gospel narratives, can be a deep and often surprising spiritual resource. After returning to one's office from an encounter with a patient, or a meeting with staff and family, associations with biblical references come to mind, sometimes with, sometimes without regular meditation. It seems as if the stories and texts, studied as an academic theologian, preached upon as a parish minister, or read in Sunday school or religious education, find their way into a chaplain's thinking, resonating with challenging situations. Biblical associations can take a hermeneutical function, helping to analyse the vulnerable situation.

One day on call, I met a suffering patient who was cared for by a network of family members and highly trained professionals, but still seemed nonresponsive to treatment and noncompliant with other options. Reflecting on the situation, the story of Jesus' healing in Mark 2:1ff helped me understand the situation of the ill person, always dependent on the help of others, as spiritual crisis. As much as Jesus takes time to focus on the forgiveness of sins before the physical healing, it could be helpful to consider the psychological and spiritual situation of the patient, that excludes the patient from any activity and any sense of being related to herself and any experience of agency. Therapeutic interventions would function only if she was able to liberate herself from paralysing dependence on others and take responsibility herself.

Biblical texts can become partners of dialogue, speaking to me if I am willing to listen. Healing occurs to myself and within me trying to cope with the existential situations a chaplain is confronted with. A Christian perspective on spiritual care thus needs to understand that healing in the Christian tradition starts with the word of God in sacred texts that resonates with health-related experience in current contexts. Tracy and Michael Balboni (this volume) talk about how Bible study within a small group can deepen spiritual care skills of health professionals.

2.3 Action-reaction

Chaplains describe an interplay of action and reaction: clients react to spiritual care offers; chaplains react to spiritual needs. Concepts of health and healing have to be co-constructed by chaplains and clients along the way and throughout the pastoral care-relation through endured presence, equally accepted performance of rituals and counselling. Trust is the fundamental quality and prerequisite of chaplaincy, generated by communication skills. Action in situations of vulnerability frequently occurs in gestures of bodily affection, ritual touching, and creating space to narrate experiences of vulnerability. To overcome vulnerability as a danger to human health, chaplaincy first establishes space for the recognition and visibility of vulnerability. Rebecca Klein refers to Judith Butler and others writing: "vulnerability is not seen as disempowering but should rather be seen as a *conditio humana* empowering the subject" (Klein 2022). Healing, thus, is understood as empowerment in a state of vulnerability, de-marginalizing and creating visibility and significance.

2.4 Strategies of Action

Healthcare chaplains contribute to positive changes: they are able to support clients in their search for meaning, they 'are with' patients and family who try to deal with and stand the fragility of life, and they give access to forms of religiosity and religious groups clients are familiar with, either by providing these forms themselves or by connecting clients with the community clients feel close to. The main effect of chaplaincy in health care seems to be the possibility to adapt to vulnerability as part of a whole-person care concept. Chaplains not only help patients or other individuals in dealing with intrinsic and extrinsic contingent aspects of vulnerability, but also support institutions and organizations to adapt to vulnerable situations: this can help to make the individual and the society resilient.

A concrete way of Christian healthcare chaplains' contribution to palliative, rehabilitative, and curative support is the development of a joint language for spiritual needs, resources, and support that can be understood and used by non-theologians. Linking two different systems, chaplains are – metaphorically speaking – 'translators' between separate languages of health and healing. A common language is the basis for both an interprofessional team-approach to spiritual care (from spiritual screening to planning spiritual care intervention), involvement of pastoral care persons (cf. Roser, Aebi, and Mösli 2022), and training health professionals' spiritual care competence.

3 Professionalism as Ongoing Pilgrimage

Höfler's research describes precisely the situation of vulnerability that is at the core of Christian understanding of pastoral care. In my own experience, being constantly exposed to death, dying, and grief by being a chaplain on a palliative care ward, within outpatient paediatric palliative care, and within seniors' nursing institutions for some ten years, I found my own faith challenged several times. Asked by colleagues or friends how I was able to deal with this, I would claim that I learned the most from patients and families, sometimes simply by silently sitting at the bedside of a patient. It came close to what I conceived to be meditation in loving presence. I also found solace and inspiration by reflecting on encounters with patients and other persons I met through biblical texts. Rather late, I found that this was pretty much what Anton T. Boisen had described from his own learning experience when he demanded that pastoral training should include learning from the "living human document" as well as the written documents of faith. Since I did not practice any specific regular spiritual practice besides prayer on occasion and at the end of my day, lighting occasional candles in chapels and after a demanding contact, I considered myself as not very spiritually active.

The main test to my own spiritual practice, however, came when I changed the side from being spiritual care provider to being recipient. When my husband was diagnosed with incurable colon cancer, I found myself on the other side. In the final weeks of his life, my partner stayed on 'my palliative ward', I was assigned the role of a family member by 'my team'. I was able to connect spiritually to my partner, our friends and families, and also to my own faith – doing nothing of what I had done before, except for actively going for regular walks with our dog, a very active Jack Russell terrier (note that Jack Russell, vicar of the Church of England, was a pastor, too!). Going for extended hikes after his death and months into my grieving process, proved to be a spiritual exercise for me, accepting and understanding my bodily existence and physical experience.

More than twelve years after this, I walked on the way of St. James, making the pilgrimage to Santiago de Compostela (Roser 2021). It turned out that I found that walking as a pilgrim was 'my' spiritual practice: meeting other pilgrims and people along the way showed me that they related to me in the same way patients in the hospital related to me. I even started to find out that many of my favourite biblical narratives and texts were pilgrimage stories, deepening my hermeneutical approach. Being a pilgrim constantly confronts oneself with one's own physical, psychological, and spiritual vulnerability, one's former experiences of pain, hurt, and resilience, but also one's present situation of physical and bodily need and strength. I found other pilgrims who shared their pain and joy along the way, during meals and during pilgrims' mass, connecting me to a larger community than those physically present. Being a pilgrim, I became connected to a meaningful and healing community that is still alive. I was able to live through and with grief but experiencing myself as a Protestant pastor open to meet with pilgrims from other places and other religious traditions. Being religious myself, I was able to connect spiritually in the broadest sense of the word.

Andrea Bieler makes "Verletzliches Leben" – vulnerable life – the central theme of her theology of pastoral care (Bieler 2017). Compassion and fundamental empathy mean to be available and open to the suffering of others. Pastoral care takes place between *logos* and *ethos*: while the hospital is a place of logification (or rationalization) of the *pathos*, pastoral care advocates for the experience, the inner, felt sense of the pathos related to being ill, and thus adds an ethical approach to regard the dignity and personhood of the patient. The prominent role of listening to patients' personal and specifically illness-narratives in healthcare chaplaincy is specific to this profession. Bieler combines these with the basic theological narrative of the vulnerable and affectable God, the crucified God, and even the physical phenomenology of vulnerability. Bieler operationalizes a theology of the cross, which is firmly rooted in Lutheran tradition and the dogmatic approach of Jürgen Moltmann (1974). Theology of the cross is, basically, a theology of vulnerability that understands situations of vulnerability both as situations of suffering and of opportunity, of a new opening, as spiritual growth.

4 Paradigm Shift in Chaplaincy Training: Specialized Spiritual Care Beyond the Ordained Ministry

The most challenging situation for professional Christian pastoral care within the healthcare system – for Christian chaplaincy as a whole – is the lack of human resources, persons willing to become fully trained pastoral care professionals. There are fewer and fewer students and persons who are willing to train for the ordained ministry or for other pastoral professions – an education that normally includes full academic training (more than five years at the university), two or more years within a parish context, and many months of specialized training for chaplaincy. After fulfilling their educational requirements, most of Christian theology students are needed in parish service. For those who want to become involved in healthcare chaplaincy, CPE training has to be added along the way or afterwards. But even then, the governing bodies of the church will not let them go. Openings in healthcare chaplaincy will less and less be filled with theologians needed in parish ministry. While spiritual care plays an increasingly important role in the medical and clinical world, there are not enough professional chaplains available.

Thus, it is time for new approaches. The University of Münster established a new theological Masters-program that enables healthcare professionals with a bachelor's degree or students of theology and religious studies who do not want to work within church congregations or the parish setting, to train for professional spiritual care in healthcare. The program includes CPE, although CPE is not integrated within the academic world, but is necessary for self-awareness and communication skills. This returns to the roots of the pastoral care movement when CPE was part of seminary education. The training combines knowledge of the healthcare system and its language and theological competence, including theological understanding of Christian texts and thought, thus enabling future healthcare chaplains to link both systems.

The program, hopefully, enables persons to understand themselves as Christian spiritual care providers who continue the tradition of Christian healthcare chaplaincy as pastoral care, but within a new profession especially assigned to the healthcare setting.

References

Bieler, Andrea. 2017. *Verletzliches Leben: Horizonte einer Theologie der Seelsorge.* 1st ed. Arbeiten zur Pastoraltheologie, Liturgik und Hymnologie 90. Göttingen: Vandenhoeck & Ruprecht. https://doi.org/10.13109/9783666624407.

Boisen, Anton T. 1971. *The Exploration of the Inner World: A Study of Mental Disorder and Religious Experience.* Pennsylvania: University of Pennsylvania Press.

Borneman, Tami, Betty Ferrell, and Christina M Puchalski. 2010. 'Evaluation of the FICA Tool for Spiritual Assessment'. *Journal of Pain and Symptom Management* 40 (2): 163–73.

Bourdieu, Pierre. 2023. *Die feinen Unterschiede: Kritik der gesellschaftlichen Urteilskraft.* Translated by Bernd Schwibs and Achim Russer. 29. Auflage. Suhrkamp-Taschenbuch Wissenschaft 658. Frankfurt am Main: Suhrkamp.

Bulger, Roger J, and John P McGovern, eds. 2001. *Physician and Philosopher: The Philosophical Foundation of Medicine: Essays by Dr. Edmund Pellegrino.* 1st ed. Charlottesville: Garden Jennings Publishing.

Cadge, Wendy, and Emily Sigalow. 2013. 'Negotiating Religious Differences: The Strategies of Interfaith Chaplains in Healthcare'. *Journal for the Scientific Study of Religion* 52 (1): 146–58. https://doi.org/10.1111/jssr.12008.

Carey, Lindsay B. 2012. 'Bioethical Issues and Health Care Chaplaincy in Aotearoa New Zealand'. *Journal of Religion and Health* 51 (2): 323–35. https://doi.org/10.1007/s10943-010-9368-1.

Clemm, Stephanie, Ralf J Jox, Gian Domenico Borasio, and Traugott Roser. 2015. 'The Role of Chaplains in End-of-Life Decision Making: Results of a Pilot Survey'. *Palliative and Supportive Care* 13 (1): 45–51. https://doi.org/10.1017/S1478951513000266.

EKD. 2020. *Spiritual Care durch Seelsorge. Zum Beitrag der Evangelischen Kirche im Gesundheitswesen. Eine Handreichung der Ständigen Konferenz für Seelsorge in der EKD.* Hannover: Evangelische Kirche in Deutschland. https://www.ekd.de/ekd_de/ds_doc/spiritual_care_2020.pdf.

EKD. 2023. *Wie hältst Du's mit der Kirche? Zur Bedeutung der Kirche in der Gesellschaft: Erste Ergebnisse der 6. Kirchenmitgliedschaftsuntersuchung.* Leipzig: Evangelische Verlagsanstalt.

Emlein, Günter. 2017. *Das Sinnsystem Seelsorge. Eine Studie zur Frage: Wer tut was, wenn man sagt, dass man sich um die Seele sorgt?* Göttingen: Vandenhoeck & Ruprecht.
Farr, Sebastian, Traugott Roser, and Michael Coors. 2023. 'Ethical Conflicts in Healthcare Chaplaincy: Results of an Exploratory Survey Among Protestant Chaplains in Switzerland, Germany, and Austria'. *Journal of Religion and Health* 62 (1): 130–46. https://doi.org/10.1007/s10943-022-01681-8.
Foucault, Michel. 2013. *Die Heterotopien. Der utopische Körper – zwei Radiovorträge*. Translated by Michael Bischoff. Berlin: Suhrkamp.
Gabl, Christoph. 2022. '„Das Leiden muss ein Ende haben!" Existenzielles Leiden und der Wunsch nach einem raschen Tod – ein belastendes Spannungsfeld für Palliativpatienten, Angehörige und Betreuungspersonen'. In *Assistierter Suizid: Hintergründe, Spannungsfelder und Entwicklungen*, edited by Angelika Feichtner, Ulrich Körtner, Rudolf Likar, Herbert Watzke, and Dietmar Weixler, 203–16. Berlin, Heidelberg: Springer. https://doi.org/10.1007/978-3-662-64347-1_22.
Heller, Birgit. 2014. 'Spiritualität versus Religion/Religiosität?' In *Spiritualität und Spiritual Care. Orientierungen und Impulse*, edited by Birgit Heller and Andreas Heller, 45–68. Bern: Hogrefe.
Höfler, Nika. 2022. *Wirksamkeit von Krankenhausseelsorge: Eine qualitative Studie*. Arbeiten zur praktischen Theologie (APrTh) 88. Leipzig: Evangelische Verlagsanstalt. https://doi.org/10.5771/9783374072347.
Karle, Isolde. 2010. 'Perspektiven der Krankenhausseelsorge — Eine Auseinandersetzung mit dem Konzept des Spiritual Care'. *Wege zum Menschen* 62 (6): 537–55. https://doi.org/10.13109/weme.2010.62.6.537.
Klein, Rebecca. 2022. 'Der Ethische Sinn der Verletzlichkeit. Ein Hermeneutisch-Phänomenologischer Beitrag'. In *Moralische Dimensionen der Verletzlichkeit des Menschen. Interdisziplinäre Perspektiven auf einen anthropologischen Grundbegriff und seine Relevanz für die Medizinethik*, edited by Michael Coors, 57–84. Zürich: TVZ.
Löw, Martina. 2015. 'Raumsoziologie'. Frankfurt a. M.: Suhrkamp.
Luther, Henning. 1991. 'Leben als Fragment. Der Mythos von der Ganzheit.' *Wege zum Menschen.*
Moltmann, Jürgen. 1974. *The Crucified God: The Cross of Christ as the Foundation and Criticism of Christian Theology*. London: SCM Press.
Moos, Thorsten, Simone Ehm, Fabian Kliesch, and Julia Thiesbonenkamp-Maag. 2016. *Ethik in der Klinikseelsorge: Empirie, Theologie, Ausbildung*. Arbeiten zur Pastoraltheologie, Liturgik und Hymnologie, Band 84. Göttingen Bristol, CT, U.S.A: Vandenhoeck & Ruprecht.
Nauer, Doris. 2010. *Spiritual Care statt Seelsorge?* Stuttgart: Kohlhammer.
Nolan, Steve. 2011. *Spiritual Care at the End of Life: The Chaplain as a 'Hopeful Presence'*. 1st ed. London: Jessica Kingsley Publishers.
Nolan, Steve, Philip Saltmarsh, and Carlo Leget. 2011. 'Spiritual Care in Palliative Care: Working towards an EAPC Task Force'. *European Journal of Palliative Care* 18:86–89.
Paal, Piret, Eckhard Frick, Traugott Roser, and Guy Jobin. 2017. 'Expert Discussion on Taking a Spiritual History'. *Journal of Palliative Care* 32 (1): 19–25. https://doi.org/10.1177/0825859717710888.
Peng-Keller, Simon. 2020. 'Spiritual Care: Grundgestalten, Leitmodelle und Entwicklungsperspektiven: Spiritual Care: Basic Forms, Guiding Models and Perspectives for Development'. *Spiritual Care* 9 (2): 127–35. https://doi.org/10.1515/spircare-2019-0078.
Peng-Keller, Simon. 2023. *Vom Wunder heilsamer Gegenwart: Biblisches Erzählen vom Neuwerden.* 1st ed. Würzburg: Echter.
Peng-Keller, Simon, Michael Balboni, Tracy Balboni, Annette Haußmann, Trace Haythorn, Pascal Mösli, David Neuhold, et al. 2025. 'Spiritual Care at the Crossroads: An Ecumenical White Paper

on the Future of Christian Healthcare Chaplaincy'. *Journal of Religion and Health*, February. https://doi.org/10.1007/s10943-025-02255-0.

Puchalski, Christina M, Robert Vitillo, Sharon K Hull, and Nancy Reller. 2014. 'Improving the Spiritual Dimension of Whole Person Care: Reaching National and International Consensus'. *Journal of Palliative Medicine* 17 (6): 642–56. https://doi.org/10.1089/jpm.2014.9427.

Roser, Traugott. 2021. *¡Hola! Bei Kilometer 410. Mit allen Sinnen auf dem Jakobsweg*. Göttingen: Vandenhoeck & Ruprecht.

Roser, Traugott, Renata Aebi, and Pascal Mösli. 2022. 'Indikationenset für Seelsorge: Entwicklung eines Instruments für interprofessionelles Spiritual Care nach der Delphi-Methodik'. *Spiritual Care* 11 (3): 264–74. https://doi.org/10.1515/spircare-2022-0013.

Saunders, Cicely, and David Clark. 2006. *Cicely Saunders: Selected Writings 1958—2004*. Oxford, UK: Oxford University Press. https://doi.org/10.1093/acprof:oso/9780198570530.001.0001.

Sekretariat der Deutschen Bischofskonferenz. 2022. *In der Seelsorge schlägt das Herz der Kirche — Wort der Deutschen Bischöfe zur Seelsorge*. Die Deutschen Bischöfe 110. Bonn: Sekretariat der Deutschen Bischofskonferenz.

Taylor, Carol, and Robert Dell'Oro. 2006. *Health and Human Flourishing: Religion, Medicine, and Moral Anthropology*. Washington, DC: Georgetown University Press.

John Swinton

What Does Spiritual Healing Mean?

Abstract: The concept of spiritual healing is multifaceted and complex, with spirituality being diversely defined throughout the literature. The chapter suggests that the lack of a universal definition is not a sign of meaninglessness, but rather an indication of the complexity and socially constructed nature of spiritual experiences. Spirituality is presented as a quest to address four existential questions: Who am I? Where do I come from? Where am I going? And why? These questions gain prominence in the face of illness and suffering, and have traditionally been answered within the frameworks of world religions. In the post-religious, highly individualised Western society, spirituality has evolved into a more personal and less communally shared pursuit. Individuals seek answers to life's bigger questions through personal hopes, desires, and cultural expectations, rather than through religious narratives. The chapter considers spirituality as a generic term, not tied to any specific religion or belief system, but rather a broad concept that can encompass various forms of expression and individual searches for meaning. The concept of "relational consciousness" as defined by David Hay and Rebecca Nye proposes an innate human predisposition toward spiritual experience, observable in the unadulterated spirituality of children. Their qualitative research supports the hypothesis that humans are hard-wired for spirituality, a sense of awe, and wonder, suggesting that spirituality may be a universal, generic human need rather than merely a cultural artifact. The chapter contrasts the impact of cultural milieu on the nature of spirituality, comparing collectivist cultures with the individualised Western perspective. In the West, spiritual needs and experiences are often centred around the self, focusing on personal meaning and self-actualisation.

1 Introduction

Spiritual healing, in this cultural context, is the process by which individuals find satisfying answers to spiritual questions independently of external religious influences. The chapter explores the challenges Christian chaplains may face in this secular, individualistic spiritual landscape. The relational nature of the Christian God and the interdependent community it advocates stand in stark contrast to the individualistic approach to spirituality prevalent in the West. Chaplains, formed by Christian narratives, may need to adjust and set aside fundamental as-

https://doi.org/10.1515/9783112205839-010

sumptions of their spiritual formation to provide effective spiritual care within this new context. The chapter emphasises the importance of recognising the cultural and individual nuances of spirituality in healthcare. It highlights the need for spiritual care that respects the personal spiritual journey of each individual, while acknowledging the potential for spiritual dissonance in caregivers. The exploration of a generic, innate spiritual need opens a conversation on how healthcare providers, particularly chaplains, can navigate the complexities of spiritual healing in a culturally sensitive and authentic manner.

2 The Complexities of Spirituality

The question of what spirituality is, and what 'spiritual healing' looks like, is complex. As one reads through the voluminous literature on spirituality and healthcare, one is struck by the diversity of ways in which the term 'spirituality' is defined and understood (Jastrzębski 2022; Gall, Malette, and Guirguis-Younger 2011) This could be interpreted as indicative of the meaninglessness of the term (Paley 2008). If there is no single definition, then how can it be meaningful or useful? There is a degree of apparently obvious logic in such a concern. However, there is another way in which we might understand the plurality of definitions.[1] The diversity of definitions of spirituality indicates the complexity of the experience, and the significance of the social context for the ways in which it is constructed. We might think of spirituality as relating to the desire to answer four key questions:
1. Who am I?
2. Where do I come from?
3. Where am I going to?
4. Why?

These four key existential questions come into particular prominence when we face illness and suffering.[2] They also feed into broader, more theological ques-

1 For a development of this suggestion in a slightly different direction, see Swinton and Pattison (2010).

2 A criticism of these four existential questions could be that while they capture timeless themes, their articulation leans into modern Western philosophy. They assume an individualistic perspective on spirituality that may not resonate across all cultures. Some communities define identity primarily through group belonging rather than individual search. This, in my opinion is a fair criticism. However, as the conversations around spirituality and health within the literature tend to be implicitly Western, using these questions is appropriate for the social context into

tions of meaning purpose and theodicy, such as: What is the meaning of life? What is the point? Why is their evil and suffering? Why do bad things happen to good people?[3] Traditionally, such questions have been answered by the various world religions. However, in an (arguably) post-religious and highly individualised social context such as is found in the Western world, the answers to these kinds of questions emerges from other sources. Within such a cultural milieu, spirituality is assumed to be a *personal* rather than a shared, communal thing. The ways in which such questions are answered is not through religious narratives or shared consensus. Rather, the questions are answered according to people's own personal desires, hopes and expectations for their lives. Put slightly differently, spirituality tends to mirror closely cultural assumptions about, freedom, autonomy, choice and the elevation of the voice of the individual.

This leads to answers to these kinds of questions being found in generic rather than religious ways. By 'generic' I mean that spirituality in this form is not tied to religion or any formal system of belief. Rather, it is a free-floating entity that relates to a group of similar things, but not to any particular thing. We might compare it to certain forms of medication which are manufactured as generic and then branded by companies. Or, Jazz, which is a generic musical style that includes a wide range of musical styles. Spirituality in the cultural mode relates to a core set of needs and experiences that are captured in the kind of questions I've highlighted above, but which are then given flesh in various forms as people work spirituality into the complexities of their lives. People's spiritual needs and experiences are personal, but they are also, as I have suggested, deeply shaped by the expectations of culture. In collectivist cultures which stress the importance of community, spirituality focuses on relationships and community. In individualised cultures such as those found in the West,[4] spiritual needs revolve around individuals. The focus is on *my* meaning, *my* purpose, *my* hope and so forth. Spirituality thus tends to be viewed as a mode of self-actualisation, with spiritual care relating to ensuring that individuals can find answers to spiritual questions with-

which I am speaking, although bearing in mind their cultural boundedness and relativity is very important. I will try to emphasise the nature of this cultural boundedness as the essay moves on.

3 For a deeper exploration of theodicy and pastoral care see Swinton (2007).

4 By "The West" I refer to Europe, Scandinavia, The United States, Canada, Australia, New Zealand and those countries deeply influenced by post Enlightenment thinking. Post-Brexit Britain remains geographically a part of Europe despite its apparent desire to distance itself from the European Union.

out the overt imposition of external influences. Spiritual healing emerges as these questions are satisfactorily answered.[5]

This relatively new way of thinking about spirituality inevitably creates a contrast and potential tension for Christian chaplains, whose spiritual formation occurs within a quite different kind of spirituality. The Christian God is relational (Volf 1997). The trinity – God as three persons in one – informs us that sitting at the heart of the universe is a relational God who calls humans into relationship and holds them there with bonds of love. From creation onwards, it is made clear that "It is not good that humans should be alone (Genesis 2:18). The culmination of the gospel is the revelation of the solidarity of Jesus with human beings (Eastman 2022) and the formation of a community – the Body of Christ (1 Corinthians 12:27) – within which the disciples of Jesus are deeply interconnected and dependent on one another. Indeed, as we shall see later in this chapter, the whole of creation is deeply interconnected. In order to function within a spiritual context which assumes spirituality to be individualistic and generic, chaplains formed by the Christian narrative, have to adjust and put to one side basic assumptions of their own formation, in order effectively to offer spiritual care. This potentially creates spiritual dissonance for the chaplain and holds the potential for troublesome inauthenticity, something that we will return to in a few moments.

It will be helpful now to go a little deeper into the significance and texture of generic spirituality. The question we will address now is: *is there any evidence to suggest that human beings have generic spiritual needs, or is it merely a cultural preference?*

3 On Being Human: Relational Consciousness

Several years ago, my former colleague at the university of Aberdeen, David Hay, along with his collaborator Rebecca Nye, coined the term *relational consciousness* to define the innate nature of spirituality. In their book *The Spirit of the Child (2006),* Hay and Nye present a fascinating piece of qualitative research designed to explore children's spirituality. They worked with the hypothesis put forward by the biologist Alistair Hardy, that human beings are hard-wired for spiritual experience (Hardy 1976). If this hypothesis was true, the place we might see it most clearly is in the lives of children, before their spirituality was overly influ-

5 That is not to suggest that Western people are not also drawn to religion and community. It is simply to point out that in a rapidly secularising social context, religion as a source of community and spiritual fulfilment is not the norm for many people.

enced by their culture. In their research, they discovered that children had a natural sense of awe and wonder, a fascination with mystery and a desire to reach out and relate to others and to the transcendent. They named this natural desire to reach out and contact others at a relational level, *relational consciousness*. This mode of consciousness, they argued, is in all of us for evolutionary purposes. Everyone has a built-in spirituality. Their argument is that there is a core universal spirituality which manifests itself in various forms, one of which is religion. Religion is a manifestation of relational consciousness, but not the only manifestation.[6] This way of thinking sits well with the idea of generic spirituality.

There are, of course, problems with this perspective. For example, theories of relational consciousness are arguably rooted in particular Western psychological frameworks that may not translate cross-culturally (Christopher et al. 2014). This is a fair concern. Hay and Nye do no intercultural work. Whilst this can't be discussed here, there is a need critically to consider this theory across cultures. Again, we might wonder if in arguing for a single source of spirituality, Haye and Nye end up ontologising spirituality in a way that reduces it to nothing other than a function of the brain. Again, this is a fair concern. However, in this case, Hay does address such concerns. Hay, who was a committed Roman Catholic, does not intend for relational consciousness to be viewed in reductive terms as nothing-but brain activity. The general theory of evolution that runs through all of his work runs something like this: the eye develops because there is something to see, the ear develops because there is something to hear, and spirituality develops because there is something beyond the self to relate to. His idea of relational consciousness does argue for a universal spirituality, but it does not in any sense exclude the possibility of God or the significance of religion.

Positively, as embodied relational creatures, we need not be surprised to find that our spirituality is hard-wired into us. We need our bodies to experience anything and everything in the world. So, while Hay and Nye's theory has its difficulties, the idea that we have an innate spirituality which is seeking expression, sits reasonably comfortable with generic spirituality, and to an extent, Cristian spirituality as I have briefly outlined it above.

---

6 This of course is slightly problematic theologically insofar as it takes us back to the idea of that the manifestation of spirituality as a personal choice. Nevertheless, if it is the case that we are made in the image of a relational God and designed to relate (see later in this chapter), it is not particularly controversial to suggest that that relationality is present in all people even though it may not be directed towards God in the way that the Genesis account indicates that it should be. Relational consciousness might be considered the mechanism that enables relationality, which finds its true focus in God, but in an arguably post-religious Western context, manifests itself in various forms.

There are two important consequences that emerge from Hay and Nye's theory. Firstly, whilst humans have an inherent relational consciousness – an intrinsic desire to connect with that which lies outside of us – the assumed norms of Western culture have a different view of human beings. We are taught from early on that we are discrete individuals who may choose to join with others, but whose true state is as self-defining individuals. The idea of altruism, community, religion, and the centrality of relationships are all considered optional. Hay and Nye point out that this kind of individualism is an *unnatural* way for human beings to live. This leads to frustration, confusion, isolation and ultimately to problems that emerge from the fragmentation of our natural desire for communion. Importantly, they suggest that the ways in which we educate our children can serve to despiritualise them. Alongside of being culturally educated to assume the normality of individualism, children are taught a certain way of thinking about what is true and what is not true. They are taught that science, mathematics, empiricism are the only real ways to find truth. Things like spirituality, love, ethics, morality etc. are assumed to be optional and personal rather than communal choices. So, the system of education we assume to be helping children thrive is actually serving to despiritualise them in profound ways. A question to ponder is whether our secular healthcare services are set up in a way that despiritualises people, that is minimises, excludes of fails to notice people's existential questions when they emerge in times of crisis.

Secondly, the underlying suggestion is that *secularism is a myth.* Elsewhere, Hay argues that:

> Secularism led to the privatisation of the sacred, and that is what we find in society today and what is referred to as 'spirituality'. Many are alienated from churches because they are products of a secular system that has devalued public worship, and focused spiritual life in the human subject. This has weakened religion in the public sphere and intensified spiritual longing in the private sphere. It is a paradoxical situation, so that as formal religions continue to decline, interest in spirituality is skyrocketing (Hay and Hunt 2000, 846).

Individualism is a myth. Secularism is a myth which has been created by Western culture and which now appears 'normal' but is, in fact, significantly abnormal as is indicated by rising rates of loneliness and existential homelessness, depression, anxiety, combined with a search for spirituality and connection (Klussman et al. 2020).

Hay and Nye's suggestions raise important questions regarding healthcare and spiritual healing. If they are correct, chaplains and other healthcare professionals need to be on the lookout for the emergence of relational consciousness as it emerges in times of trauma and strife. An example will help draw out the importance of this.

It is worth noting that recent developments in developmental psychology and related disciplines provide further empirical support for the claim that relationality lies at the heart of human identity and experience. In particular, the field of interpersonal neurobiology, as developed by scholars such as Daniel Siegel, offers significant insights into the way human beings are biologically and neurologically wired for relationships (Siegel 1999). Siegel's integrative work demonstrates that relational connection is not simply a psychological preference but is fundamental to the development of neural integration, emotional regulation, and identity formation (Siegel 2020). While this chapter does not seek to provide a detailed psychological analysis, it is clear that these emerging scientific perspectives resonate with and arguably reinforce the theological claim that human beings are inherently relational creatures, created to flourish in connection with God, others, and creation. This alignment between theology and interpersonal neurobiology opens up rich possibilities for future interdisciplinary exploration within healthcare chaplaincy.

4 Breast Cancer and Relational Consciousness

A number of years ago myself and my colleague Professor Steve Heys, an oncologist at Aberdeen Royal Infirmary, specialising in breast cancer, carried out a piece of research designed so see if the idea of relational consciousness has any kind of empirical basis that might be significant for clinical care. We interviewed women during their first year after receiving the diagnosis of breast cancer. The intention was to see whether their experience of encountering a breast cancer diagnosis stimulated the emergence of relational consciousness. As we talked with these women, it became clear that an inherent sense of relationality did indeed come to the fore as they worked their way through the complexities of receiving and living with this diagnosis.

We discovered that there were three dimensions to the women's experience, the first was a movement inwards wherein they withdrew into themselves in order to make sense of this new identity as a 'breast cancer sufferer.' When a person receives a diagnosis of cancer, it changes their identity in profound ways. Before the diagnosis, you were just an ordinary person. Now they are a 'cancer sufferer,' with all that goes with such a change of identity. Cancer is an identity that you can't really get rid of. It is impossible to get away from this new identity. Even if you are considered clear of the disease, it is framed as being 'in remission.' The turn inwards was a recognition of this as women wrestled with the fact that many of the certainties they had previously held about life – future, family, careers – were now challenged by the uncertainty their new identity brought to them. The movement inwards was lonely and marked by a sense of disconnection from self and others. The big questions – who am I? Where do I come from? Where am I going? Why? – were high on these women's agenda.

The second movement was outwards. Having wrestled with the implications of their new identity, eventually, they turned their thoughts outwards. At this stage, the women began to notice relational connections they had previously overlooked. They began to reconnect with old friends and networks; to have a heightened experience of their love for family and friends. They began to sense they were caught up in a series of vital relational networks which had always been there but had been hidden from notice because of the busyness of life. This was in line with the suggestion that they were discovering or re-encountering their relational consciousness.

The third movement, for some, was upwards. Some women began to realise the importance of finding or strengthening their connection with God. They recognised the importance of their social relationships, but in order to answer the questions that came to mind, they needed a wider, more transcendent canvas to make sense of their experiences. God became a vital dimension of their relational network.

Through the study, it became clear that there was an emergence of relational consciousness as people encountered the trauma of cancer. For some, the search for relationship was generic, for others it was religious. It was also clear that spiritual care was different in each of these phases of a person's illness. In times of trouble or stress, this natural spirituality will come into play in ways that are important but easily overlooked. The key to spiritual care was to be sensitised to the experiences that people went through in their different phases, and to offer care based on people's expressed needs.

5 Managing Pluralism

The idea of generic spirituality, as I have outlined and developed it here, has much to offer to the practice of healthcare. It is not, however, without its problems and challenges. There is a tension with regard to the idea of generic spirituality and generic chaplaincy that is worth considering. Earlier I indicated the ways in which culture and context work themselves out in terms of the shape and form of spirituality within a Western context. I highlighted individualism as a key aspect of the construction of spirituality. However, the ways in which societies are becoming much more pluralistic and multicultural presents an interesting challenge to the conversation around generic spirituality.

Chaplain Duncan MacLaren points to a tension within the United Kingdom, wherein the National Health Service, in Scotland and England, deal with issues around pluralism differently (MacLaren 2021). In Scotland, the aim seems to be to keep religion firmly out of public healthcare. This has led to the development of "generic" chaplains (Cobb 2005) – chaplains who work independently of the specifics of religious or belief identity, requiring the "de-emphasising of one's own particularity" (Kotva 1998, 226, in MacLaren 2021, 18). In England, the focus has been on developing multi faith perspectives within which "diversity is acknowledged and celebrated." (MacLaren 2021, 18; see also Swift, this volume). These two options lie at either end of what has been termed the "particularist-universalist" continuum (Liefbroer, Ganzevoort, and Olsman 2019, 244–60; in MacLaren 2021, 28).

MacLaren is unconvinced by either model. The generic model urges chaplains to put their own beliefs and formation to one side and simply care for the generic needs of patients, with the religious needs being left to local clergy and religious leaders. In practice, this approach is impractical – would an Anglican chaplain spend hours finding a local clergy person to baptise a baby rather than doing it themselves? – and unhealthy – the spiritual formation of the chaplain is crucial for their own well-being and the effective practice of spiritual care.

The multi-faith model is also problematic insofar as a focus on religion risks missing the spiritual needs of the non-religious:

> . . . the visibly religious presentation of the multi-faith model arguably perpetuates the perception among clinical staff that chaplaincy teams are mostly there to provide religious care for the faithful, rather than spiritual care for all – a perception that can lead to inequitable access to spiritual care for those of no specific faith or belief (MacLaren 2021, 29)

MacLaren offers a third way, wherein the chaplain takes seriously their own spiritual formation as it emerges from the wisdom tradition of their faith. Whilst the roots of their formation may remain invisible in terms of practice, a focus on formation, tradition and wisdom enables the chaplain to remain authentic, and to retain their integrity within a complex pluralistic healthcare context. This way avoids reducing the richness of chaplaincy and allows the wisdom of tradition to inform their practices in constructive ways. He urges chaplains to claim and live into their identity as *professionals*:

> . . . it might be more accurate to refer to ourselves as "professional" – a deliberate double-entendre, which picks up the older meaning of the word, relating to religious vows. Professional chaplains are those who bring their whole selves to their work, including the "profes-

> sion" of their beliefs and practices. The chaplain who is called to the bedside of a dying person in the small hours of the morning will, at best, turn up "whole." Whatever their faith or belief tradition – Christian, Buddhist, Humanist, etc. they will bring a view of what it means to be human that has been formed within their own spiritual "modality." In this way, they are being "professional" in both senses of the word – both safe and effective, and resourced by the wisdom tradition in which they have been formed. Perhaps we are only being fully professional when we integrate both these senses in our practice. By doing so, we may open a way to offer spiritual care with integrity in the heart of a plural health service (MacLaren 2021, 38).

My sense is that MacLaren's suggestion is wise. It is possible to recognise the spiritual needs of all people without stripping the chaplain of their spiritual roots and placing them in a position where vital healing resources are overlooked or downgraded. The generic approach orients us to the fact that all people have a spirituality. MacLaren's position enables us to take seriously our personal formative beliefs as a crucial aspect of caring for the wider spiritual needs of all of the people we seek to care for. The generic and the religious may stand in tension, but they need not be seen as being in opposition. In the light of MacLaren's suggestion, the question we will turn to now is: *What kind of spiritual wisdom informs Christian chaplaincy, and what difference might it make for practice?*

6 Chaplaincy and Christian Wisdom

A Christian model of chaplaincy based on Christian wisdom takes seriously the idea that all people have a spirituality, alongside of the important observation that religion matters in both theory and practice. A central aspect of Christian wisdom in a healthcare context relates to the fact that it begins with a different understanding of health, which results in a different understanding of healing. The World Health Organization's definition of health states that "Health is a state of complete physical, mental and social well-being and not merely the absence of disease or infirmity" (World Health Organization 2025). The aspirational goals of this definition are to promote holistic health and high standards globally (Peng-Keller, Winiger, and Rauch 2022). The well-intended motivations of the definition provide helpful context. However, the WHO definition sets an extremely high bar for health as "complete physical, mental and social well-being." This maximalist standard is likely unrealistic. Likewise, the focus on "absence of disease" promotes a negative orientation toward health rather than a positive model of flourishing. This in turn may reinforce a reductionist view of medicine as curing disease rather than promoting holistic wellness. This is a maximalist concept which sets the bar for health at an unachievably high level. According to this way of thinking about health, *we are all ill*, as none of us reach the maximum implied by the definition. If health is the complete physical, mental and social well-being, then medicine should be ensuring we achieve that. This is the seedbed for assumptions that health has to do with the absence of illness and distress. Nevertheless, the desire to promote holistic health and high standards globally, is admirable if we take seriously the WHO definitions' emphasis on health being "not merely the absence of disease or infirmity." These two dimensions of the definition resonate in important ways with a theological perspective on health.

7 Health as *Shalom*

The bible does not have a word that is equivalent to a biomedical view of health as the absence of illness. Instead, the bible focuses on the term *shalom*, which means peace: peace within ourselves, between ourselves and others, peace with creation, and ultimately peace with God. Sitting at the heart of the term shalom is justice, righteousness, right relationship with God (Wilkinson 1998). To be healthy is to be in right relationship with God. Everything else springs from this core relationship. Within *shalom*, it is not necessary for someone to be cured in order for them to be healthy and healed. Health is not perceived as the absence of the symptoms of illness. It is marked by the presence of God and the presence of others, even in the midst of illness.

The "others" in that statement is important. Unlike the generic model of spirituality discussed previously, which I have suggested does have some contextual utility, Christian spirituality is always corporate and communal. We are the Body of Christ; persons-in-relation, bound together by bonds of love and mutuality. Such love is not simply aimed internally at the Body. It reaches out into the world God so loved that he gave us Jesus (John 3:16), the one in whom all things are being reconciled (Colossians 1:19–20). Whilst shalom-as-health might at one level seem exclusive – what about people who are not Christian – in terms of practice and formation, it does at least two things. Firstly, it enables the chaplain to reframe his or her understanding of health away from simply pushing against illness, towards connection even in the midst of illness. Ideally (from a faith perspective), this connection is with God. However, that connection can also come through the Christian chaplain as a representative of God and fellow traveller who is correspondingly made in the image of God. Shalom locates the chaplain as a relational conduit focused on facilitating connection with the person before them. Secondly, it offers a different understanding of spiritual healing. In this way of thinking, healing is not defined by the absence of illness or distress, but by the presence of God, manifested in the presence and demeanour of the chaplain. Spiritual healing is thus seen not to relate purely to curing, but rather with connecting. It is for example, possible to be dying of some kind of terminal illness and to be healed even if cure is not a possibility. A person may not be cured, but within this understanding of health, they can find healing. It is as we are helped to find our connections with God and with one another that we begin to discover what it means to be healed.

The theological richness of *shalom* as a vision of human flourishing has been explored extensively by scholars such as Nicholas Wolterstorff (2004, 70), who describes *shalom* not merely as the absence of conflict or illness, but as the presence of justice, relational harmony, and a right ordering of life before God. In this light, spiritual healing is not limited to cure or the restoration of physical health; rather, it involves enabling people, even in conditions of suffering, illness, and dying to experience themselves as beloved, connected, and embraced within the sustaining relationships of God and community. Healthcare chaplaincy, at its best, participates in this work of *shalom by* creating spaces where individuals can rediscover their relational identity and dignity, irrespective of their physical prognosis.

8 Developing a Christian Spirituality for Chaplains

The model of generic spirituality, and the idea of relational consciousness, allows us to assume that all people have a spirituality and that all people desire to relate at a temporal and a transcendent level. We might think of this theologically in terms of the image of God in all human beings. Precisely what the image of God is, has been the subject of debate and controversy throughout Christian history (Cortez 2017). A reflection on the Genesis account of creation is revealing. God breathes His spirit (*nephesh)* into all creation (Genesis 2:7). Phenomenologically there is no difference between humans and other creatures. The difference is that Gods chooses to talk to Adam. The image is revealed in God's relationship with Adam and the profound statement that it is not good for humans to be alone (Genesis 2:18). Human beings are by design persons-in-relation. It is therefore not surprising that we might discover something like relational consciousness as a mechanism for connection between humans and between humans and God.

There is another dimension to the image of God that has great importance for chaplaincy. In Colossians 1:15, Paul tells us: "The Son is the image of the invisible God, the firstborn over all creation." Jesus is the image of God. As we look at

Jesus, so we see something of God among us. The image of God thus has the potential to work in two ways in the work of chaplains. At the general level, it provides a basic caring principle which allows the chaplain to embrace all people, as all of us are made in the image of God and worthy of love and care. At another level, it reminds us of the Christ-centred and indeed cosmic nature of our work as Christian chaplains, as we participate with Jesus in the redemption of creation. As bearers of God's *shalom*, we are participants in the redemption of the world through the work of Jesus. This kind of deep Christian wisdom, even if it is not formally articulated, enables wise practice that includes both the generic and the specific aspects of people's spiritual lives.

9 What is Spiritual Healing?

In moving towards a conclusion to this chapter, we can begin to work through some aspects of what spiritual healing is. In the light of what has been discussed thus far, we might describe some of the key features of spiritual healing in this way:

> Spiritual healing has to do with the connection and reconnection of human relationships both temporal and divine. It is brought about through relationships, practices and interventions which enable individuals and systems to find and strengthen connections in any given situation. Spiritual healing is not determined by the ability to cure ailments. Rather, spiritual healing relates to enabling people to hold on to relationships with self, others and God, amidst the complexities of a person's life.

This kind of spiritual healing need not be viewed as something apart from medical healing. In order for chaplains to become spiritual healers who carry the vision of *shalom* into the healthcare context, it is necessary that the chaplain bears within them both approaches to healthcare. In her book *Theology and Pastoral Counselling*, the pastoral theologian Deborah van Deusen Hunsinger sets out to discern the role of theology in deep therapy (Hunsinger 1995) using the pattern of the incarnation and the assertion that in the body of Jesus, humanity and the Divine are one, she argues that the role of the therapist is to hold within herself two models of therapy, one which is informed by psychology, the other by theology. They cannot and should not be separated. The ground of their consolidation is the body of the therapist. This Christological model provides a useful way of thinking about how the chaplain can bring together the two models of health discussed in this paper, firstly within their own bodies/practices, and from thereon into the system more generally. The chaplain holds in tension the need for medicine and medical healing and the importance of spiritual and relational reconnection. The chaplain recognises the tensions that emerge from caring in a context that often self-identifies as secular and can be profoundly individualistic, and the recognition that human beings are inherently relational, and that connection may be their primary need in any given situation.

10 Conclusion: Towards Holistic Spiritual Healing

This exploration of healthcare chaplaincy and spiritual healing has illuminated some key tensions in conceptualizing spirituality in modern healthcare contexts. The emergence of generic, individualistic notions of spirituality clash with religious traditions that view spiritual identity as rooted in community. Biomedical models focus on curing bodily ailments, while theological frameworks like shalom emphasise holistic wellbeing and right relationships. These complexities underline the challenges facing chaplains aiming to provide spiritual care in a pluralistic setting. Integration of disparate perspectives is possible through a vision of chaplaincy that honours both common spiritual needs and the diverse religious formations of caregivers. Embracing their identity and traditions allows chaplains to offer authentic presence. Concepts like relational consciousness and the image of God provide anchors for compassionately responding to all people's spirituality.

Spiritual healing is defined not by cure, but by enabling connections to self, others, and the transcendent. This requires chaplains to advocate for nurturing spiritual health amidst medical priorities. As "prophets of the spiritual," chaplains can ensure healthcare systems support meaning and purpose. Drawing on theological wisdom, social science, and evidence of spiritual care's benefits, chaplains can act as cultural brokers–building trust, easing tensions, and spurring change. We might sum up this chaplaincy role as relating to the chaplain becoming a cultural broker. The healthcare system contains many different cultures – those of patients, families, doctors, nurses, administrators, and more. Each brings diverse perspectives on health, healing, spirituality, and what matters most. When these cultures clash or fail to understand one another, problems arise. Patients may feel uncared-for in body, mind, or spirit. Staff can become frustrated and dismissive. Organisational priorities may neglect deeper human needs. If such cultural tensions are to be relieved, there is a need for cultural brokerage. The aim of the culture broker is to help individuals and systems recognise the importance of spiritual healing as the basis for all their activities. The cultural broker bridges, links and mediates between various groups of people with a view to reducing conflict and enhancing healing. As culture brokers, chaplains can build trust and promote practices that reconnect patients and staff to life's meaning and purpose. They can draw on theological wisdom, social science, and evidence on spiritual care's positive impacts to spur change. Culture brokers are intermediaries who move between individuals, patients, healthcare professionals and, in this case, healthcare systems. This, it seems to me, is a potentially powerful role for the chaplain. Cultural brokerage alongside of Christian wisdom and a desire to enable spiritual healing present the chaplain with a unique role that takes seriously his or her spiritual formation but allows them to bring haling and reconciliation to a broad range of people.

It is important to clarify that the metaphor of the chaplain as a 'cultural broker' does not imply an unrealistic functional capacity or an idealised omnipresence within healthcare systems. Given the current pressures on healthcare chaplaincy, including limited staffing and increasing demands, such an interpretation would be both impractical and theologically misleading. Rather, this image seeks to highlight the distinctive vocation of chaplains in inhabiting and navigating spaces of complexity, pluralism, and existential need not through professional omnipotence but via theological rootedness, pastoral presence, and relational attentiveness. The brokered space is fragile, contingent, and reliant on the chaplain's capacity for humility and hospitality. Theological integrity necessitates an honest reckoning with these limitations.

In the end, spiritual healing in healthcare is about reconciliation – of competing worldviews, of bodies and spirits, of life's uncertainties. By bridging divides, chaplains manifest God's shalom and enable whole-person care. Though the path is complex, chaplains have a unique opportunity to reunite and restore what is broken. May we respond to this calling with wisdom, compassion, and hope.

References

Christopher, John Chambers, Dennis C Wendt, Jeanne Marecek, and David M Goodman. 2014. 'Critical Cultural Awareness: Contributions to a Globalizing Psychology'. *The American Psychologist* 69 (7): 645–55. https://doi.org/10.1037/a0036851.

Cobb, Mark. 2005. 'The Hospitals' Spirit and the Generic Chaplain'. *Journal of Health Care Chaplaincy* 14 (1): 7–15.

Cortez, Marc. 2017. *ReSourcing Theological Anthropology: A Constructive Account of Humanity in the Light of Christ*. Grand Rapids, Michigan: Zondervan Academic.

Eastman, Susan. 2022. 'Christian Experience and Paul's Logic of Solidarity: The Spiral Structure of Romans 5–8'. *The Biblical Annals* 12 (2): 233–53. https://doi.org/10.31743/biban.13513.

Gall, Terry Lynn, Judith Malette, and Manal Guirguis-Younger. 2011. 'Spirituality and Religiousness: A Diversity of Definitions'. *Journal of Spirituality in Mental Health*, July. https://www.tandfonline.com/doi/abs/10.1080/19349637.2011.593404.

Hardy, Alister Clavering. 1976. *The Biology of God: A Scientist's Study of Man the Religious Animal*. First Edition. New York: Taplinger Pub. Co.
Hay, David, and Kate Hunt. 2000. 'Is Britain's Soul Waking up?' *The Tablet*, June.
Hay, David, and Rebecca Nye. 2006. *The Spirit of the Child: Revised Edition*. Revised ed. London: Jessica Kingsley Publishers.
Hunsinger, Deborah van Deusen. 1995. *Theology and Pastoral Counseling: A New Interdisciplinary Approach*. Standard Edition. Grand Rapids, Mich: Wm. B. Eerdmans-Lightning Source.
Jastrzębski, Andrzej K. 2022. 'The Challenging Task of Defining Spirituality'. *Journal of Spirituality in Mental Health* 24 (2): 113–31. https://doi.org/10.1080/19349637.2020.1858734.
Klussman, Kristine, Austin Lee Nichols, Julia Langer, and Nicola Curtin. 2020. 'Connection and Disconnection as Predictors of Mental Health and Wellbeing'. *International Journal of Wellbeing* 10 (2). https://doi.org/10.5502/ijw.v10i2.855.
Kotva, Joseph J. 1998. 'Hospital Chaplaincy As Agapeic Intervention'. *Christian Bioethics*, December, 257–75.
Liefbroer, Anke I, R Ruard Ganzevoort, and Erik Olsman. 2019. 'Addressing the Spiritual Domain in a Plural Society: What Is the Best Mode of Integrating Spiritual Care into Healthcare?' *Mental Health, Religion & Culture* 22 (3): 244–60.
MacLaren, Duncan. 2021. 'All Things to All People? The Integrity of Spiritual Care in a Plural Health Service'. *Health and Social Care Chaplaincy* 9 (1): 27–41. https://doi.org/10.1558/hscc.40568.
Paley, John. 2008. 'Spirituality and Nursing: A Reductionist Approach'. *Nursing Philosophy: An International Journal for Healthcare Professionals* 9 (1): 3–18. https://doi.org/10.1111/j.1466-769X.2007.00330.x.
Peng-Keller, Simon, Fabian Winiger, and Raphael Rauch. 2022. *The Spirit of Global Health: The World Health Organization and the 'Spiritual Dimension' of Health, 1946–2021*. Oxford, New York: Oxford University Press.
Siegel, Daniel J. 1999. *The Developing Mind: Toward a Neurobiology of Interpersonal Experience*. First Edition. New York: The Guilford Press.
Siegel, Daniel J. 2020. *The Developing Mind: How Relationships and the Brain Interact to Shape Who We Are*. 3rd ed. New York London: The Guilford Press.
Swinton, John. 2007. *Raging with Compassion: Pastoral Responses to the Problem of Evil*. Grand Rapids, Mich: Wiiliam B. Eerdmans Pub.
Swinton, John, and Stephen Pattison. 2010. 'Moving beyond Clarity: Towards a Thin, Vague, and Useful Understanding of Spirituality in Nursing Care'. *Nursing Philosophy* 11:226–37. https://doi.org/10.1111/j.1466-769x.2010.00450.x.
Volf, Miroslav. 1997. *After Our Likeness: The Church as the Image of the Trinity*. First edition. Grand Rapids, Mich: Wm. B. Eerdmans Publishing Co.
Wilkinson, John. 1998. *The Bible and Healing: A Medical and Theological Commentary*. Edinburgh: Handsel Press.
Wolterstorff, Nicholas. 2004. *Educating for Shalom: Essays on Christian Higher Education*. Edited by Clarence W. Joldersma and Gloria Goris Stronks. Grand Rapids, MI: Wm. B. Eerdmans-Lightning Source.
World Health Organization. 2025. 'Health and Wellbeing'. The Global Health Observatory: Explore a World of Health Data. 2025. https://www.who.int/data/gho/data/major-themes/health-and-well-being#:~:text=The%20WHO%20constitution%20states%3A%20%22Health,of%20mental%20disorders%20or%20disabilities.

Wim Smeets

Professional Competence and Autonomy of General Spiritual Caregivers in the Netherlands

Abstract: Spiritual care in the Netherlands has undergone enormous development over the last half century, closely linked to the changed worldview landscape in society. Not only do people draw from multiple sources for their spirituality, spiritual caregivers do so themselves. A new group of spiritual caregivers has emerged who cannot or do not want to receive a mission from a church or other worldview organization, but who receive a mandate from an independent council for non-institutionally bound spiritual caregivers. A case study illustrates how spiritual competency and spiritual care competency apply to these new spiritual caregivers and how they relate to their church colleagues. This development towards more autonomy is not at odds with, but is actually in line with, the development of Christian spirituality. This also has consequences for CPE as the most important further training for spiritual caregivers worldwide.

1 Introduction

In 2010, we published a book on the occasion of the farewell of a Catholic spiritual caregiver at Radboud University Medical Center (Radboudumc, Den Draak and Smeets 2010). It outlined his professional biography against the background of developments in the profession. Ries Van de Sande's development begins in his native village, where he met the local Franciscan fathers. He completes the priestly training and becomes a follower of Francis of Assisi. He is active in youth care and later becomes a chaplain in health care. It is a turbulent time for Catholicism in the Netherlands. In 1971, the Pastoral Council of all pastoral leaders in the Netherlands is held, which calls for major changes in the Catholic Church. The role of women, the role of the lay person in general, democratization and the abolition of compulsory priestly celibacy are some of the important themes that are discussed. In this climate, many priests resign and marry, in the belief that they will soon be able to continue working as married chaplains. That is what Ries does, too. He receives a mission from the bishop to work as a married chaplain.

But the tide is turning. The Dutch bishops are whistled back in Rome. New, much more conservative bishops are appointed. When Ries starts working at Rad-

https://doi.org/10.1515/9783112205839-011

boudumc, the bishop refuses to grant him a mission. The board of the Catholic university hospital is outraged and decides to give Ries an appointment, against the wishes of the bishop. For many years, Ries works as a Catholic chaplain in the hospital, including the children's wards and in the care of cancer patients. The head of the palliative care department expressly wants more attention for spirituality in the care of people in the last phase of life. But in order to be able to work well in the team, he wants Ries not to invoke pastoral secrecy. That is why he proposes a new job title: 'spiritual care consultant'. In the last years of his working life Ries works in this position.

What a development: starting as a father and ending as a 'consultant'. And yet, Ries himself sees a lot of continuity in his work. One of the authors shadows Ries during a working week. He listens a lot to people. He describes his work as follows: "Learning to see and name what the spiritual layer is in the life story of the patient. What is ultimately at stake for this woman or man? What is her or his deepest belief in life? What values and valuations emerge in the life story? How does someone deal with the situation: resigned or courageously? What life resources are being tapped? What is the meaning of everything that happens?" (den Draak and Smeets, 2010, 22). With the same conviction, he leads in prayer: "May the Eternal who is faithful to us humans, a faithfulness stronger than death, remain near you. By day and by night, in living, suffering and dying, until you are completed according to his purpose. May the Eternal be near you when you cry out: It is finished. In the name of the Eternal Father, Son, and Spirit. Amen." (den Draak and Smeets, 2010, 29).

The professional biography of this colleague shows a development from a representative of a (specific) faith community to a 'specialized health professional'. Is this a favourable or fatal development, is it coincidental – typically Dutch – or inevitable for Christian spiritual care? We will address that question in this contribution. First, we characterize spiritual care in the Dutch health care sector, against the background of developments in the field of religion and worldview in society. We then discuss a specific Dutch development, that of the recognition of general or non-denominational spiritual caregivers. We clarify what this organizational development means in concrete terms by means of an in-depth interview with a spiritual caregiver who has Catholic roots but expressly positions herself as a general spiritual caregiver. Based on this, we first reflect on the concept of spiritual competence and from there on the professional autonomy of the spiritual caregiver with a Christian inspiration. Finally, we discuss the significance of this for the further training of spiritual caregivers, particularly in clinical pastoral education.

2 Spiritual Care and Health Care: a Survey in the Netherlands

In the first large-scale study into the quality of spiritual care in the Netherlands, we examined, among other things, the goals of the profession. Spiritual care is the health care profession that has spirituality as its special domain. We define spirituality with Puchalski et al. as "a dynamic and intrinsic aspect of humanity through which persons seek ultimate meaning, purpose, and transcendence, and experience relationship to self, to family, others, community, society, nature, and the significant or sacred. Spirituality is expressed through beliefs, values, traditions, and practices" (Puchalski et al. 2009, 646).

Our belief is that the purpose of the profession is related to the goals of care as well as to goals in the domain of spirituality. The overall goal of health care is to promote people's health. The healthcare sector tries to provide quality care, both by appropriate interaction with patients and by organizing multidisciplinary collaboration, including through protocols for the process of patient care. The overall goal of spirituality is to develop meaning and the connection with oneself, others and the sacred, the relationship between human beings and God. This means that the focus of spiritual care in healthcare should be sought at the intersection of the purpose of healthcare and the purpose of spiritual care in general. After all, it is important that spiritual care is integrated into healthcare and does not remain isolated (Smeets, Gribnau, and van der Ven 2011, 99–105). The definition of the goal of spiritual care in health care is as follows: promoting the health of people by means of communication about spirituality, or: to promote spiritual health. We are by no means aiming for a 'healthification of spirituality', but it is expressed that health as a focus of care also includes a spiritual aspect in addition to a physical, psychological and social aspect. Communicating with patients about their spirituality contributes just as much to their well-being as the involvement of other disciplines.

In our research, we found that spiritual caregivers endorse the goals that we investigated. We also looked at how important spiritual caregivers consider the quality of care in contact with patients and the quality of care at the meso-level. It appears that spiritual caregivers pay particular attention to the quality of care at the micro-level and attach much less importance to protocols, the meso-level. The more emphasis spiritual caregivers place on the quality of care at the micro-level, the more they consider the specific purpose of their profession to be important. That spiritual caregivers take the perspective of the patient and develop a compassionate approach to patient's suffering influences their spiritual health (Smeets, Gribnau, and van der Ven 2011, 110). Integration of spiritual care in healthcare, by endorsing the quality aspects in relation to patients, does not lead to undermining one's own spiritual perspective of spiritual care. Our research shows just the opposite.

However, the spiritual purpose of the profession is complicated by another tendency, which comes from the social context. The sociocultural processes of secularization, deinstitutionalization and individualization have also become visible in healthcare institutions, affecting clients, staff and spiritual caregivers themselves. The ideological landscape in the Netherlands is highly secularized and has become very diverse. Christianity is still the numerically most important religion, but the percentages are dropping very fast. Yet more than half of the population is still involved in religion and spirituality: a quarter is a member of a church, a quarter is unattached spiritually or religiously (Bernts and Berghuijs 2016). A relatively new phenomenon is that of 'multiple religious belonging': the phenomenon of having a connection with more than one religion. This also takes place within the churches: almost half of the members of a church are inspired by several religions. The combination of Christianity and Buddhism is most common. Spiritual caregivers appear to be adapting to this new phenomenon. Liefbroer and Berghuijs asked spiritual caregivers for their opinion on this, and it appears that multiple religious belonging is not a problem for most of them. They also practice a form of interreligious spiritual care, in which they offer themselves as a partner for patients with a different belief. Only the rituals do they prefer to be performed by spiritual caregivers with the same conviction as the patient (Liefbroer and Berghuijs 2017).

3 Institutionally Not Endorsed Spiritual Caregivers: Ministry and Mandate

About 10 years ago, a new sector was founded within the professional association of spiritual caregivers in the Netherlands: the sector for institutionally unattached colleagues. It was the result of years of consultation between various parties involved, from the professional group itself, the study programs, the worldview communities and scientific experts. I closely followed the process from the latter point of view. As a result, spiritual caregivers who are unwilling or unable to be sent by a worldview organization are tested for their spiritual competence by an independent council. All those involved eventually agreed that a spiritual caregiver must not only have a good education but must also be authorized from the domain of worldview. The text agreed upon by the parties concerned reads as follows: "The spiritual competence of aspiring spiritual caregivers who will not or cannot be endorsed by a religious denomination or by the Humanistic Association, shall be assessed by some sort of 'Council for independent spirituality'." Endorsement or nomination by any community of values is not an option for non-denominational spiritual caregivers. Such a community does not – and by its nature cannot – exist as a formal institution. The authorities involved in setting up this arrangement were well aware that they were setting in motion something that seemed to contradict social-religious development, namely de-institutionalization and individualization. However, they were convinced that there had to be some form of supervision of the spiritual development of these new chaplains and that it could not be left to the private self-assessment of the chaplains or their clients.

There thus is a need for an alternative institution to assess the spiritual competence of non-denominational spiritual caregivers, such as a Council" (cited in Napel-Roos et al. 2021, 68). An assessment committee, consisting of a supervisor and a spiritual caregiver, assesses an assignment, which consists of writing a personal spiritual biography and the report of and reflection on an intercultural encounter (where the interlocutor has a different worldview than the spiritual caregiver). Three elements of that authorization were and are still the subject of discussion: someone must be able to show involvement in spirituality in order to subsequently be able to represent it (belonging and representing), from there the spiritual caregiver must guarantee the client's freedom to be able to express one's own spirituality at all times (the 'sanctuary function'), and someone must be able to bring spiritual sources into interaction with a client or clients (application of spiritual sources in personal attitude and professional practice). If, according to an assessment by that council, the general spiritual caregiver has provided proof of this, she or he will be given a mandate to practice the profession (Napel-Roos et al. 2021).

In the meantime, many dozens of spiritual caregivers have gone through this procedure, and the group of non-institutionalized spiritual caregivers has grown into the second-largest sector of the profession. However, that does not mean that the discussion is over. Important issues in this area remain: how deeply embedded is the spirituality of the newcomers? How is spirituality kept alive and further developed? Who can and may perform rituals in an authentic way? 'Authentic' means that spiritual caregivers do not perform rituals that they are not mandated to perform (which are reserved for office holders on behalf of a religious community), nor that they cannot support based on their own spirituality. A good example of this is creating conditions for and being present at a prayer by clients and their relatives in a meditation centre, without saying the prayers themselves if the spiritual counsellor is not religious.

General not endorsed spiritual caregivers – they call themselves also 'general spiritual caregivers' in opposition to 'denominational spiritual caregivers' – are still regarded by many colleagues as second-class spiritual caregivers; in their view the newcomers could still qualify for the classic trajectory because 'actually they are Christian or humanistic spiritual caregivers'. Conversely, among the new spiritual caregivers, there are also people who regard their colleagues with a mission from a worldview community as representatives of the past. What does not help the latter is that their number is decreasing due to retirement and limited numbers of newcomers. That brings Hetty Zock to the following conclusion: "the professional identity of the spiritual caregiver in the Netherlands is gradually changing from primarily a religious office holder endorsed by a religious/worldview community and providing religious care, to a specific health care professional specialized in meaning-making and belief systems" (Zock 2019, 16).

4 Personal Spiritual Practice and Professionality: Interview With a General Spiritual Caregiver

Anna (fictitious name) has been a spiritual caregiver for several years, with a mandate from the Council of not endorsed spiritual care. After graduating from high school, she first took a bachelor's degree in religious studies at Radboud University Nijmegen. After that, she was in doubt about which master's program she would like to follow; after the theoretical pre-education, she wanted something practical. For a moment, she considered doing teacher training, but after a conversation with a friend she opted for the master's in spiritual care. Radboud University provides one of the general training programs for spiritual caregivers in the Netherlands, so do also the University of Groningen and the Free University of Amsterdam. In addition, there are denomination-related programs, theological courses at the Protestant University (from 2024 in Utrecht) and the School of Catholic Theology (Utrecht) and the humanistic course at the University of Humanistic Studies (also in Utrecht). Finally, there are training programs for Islamic, Hindu and Buddhist spiritual care.

Anna does not consider herself a humanist and thought the theological courses were too Christian. She was not that interested in how Christianity looks at meaning. In particular, she wanted to delve into how people without a firm belief come to deal with life. When asked about her religious background, she answers that she comes from a 'Catholic nest in Brabant', the south of the Netherlands – where Catholicism is still very much present. "The church offered stability in life, I was baptized, did communion and confirmation, and we went to church once a year because of my grandmother's death, and that was about it. My parents didn't know much about religion. We didn't pray before eating, my grandpa and grandma still did. I was raised progressively and open. My parents had friends who were homosexual, and they thought it was important that this was seen as normal. We were cultural Catholics." I ask her what her current sources are, what spirituality she feels at home with. "I feel at home in a progressive Catholic environment, also called ecumenical; I would like to continue my Catholic traditions and customs. In recent years I have moved in the direction of nature religion. I am looking for how to connect the two, the Catholic and the idea of a cyclical life."

I present her the concept of 'lived spirituality': how do you keep your spirituality alive? What do you do for that? "I read a lot, I sing in a choir, connected to a monastic congregation. That choir has the status of a worldview community: we celebrate together, we discover together, I am in the text group and on the board. In addition, I go outside and like to be in nature." Another concept I present to her is 'embodied spirituality'. How does your spirituality become flesh and blood, what is the role of the body in your spirituality experience? "I have only recently become more aware of this. While singing, your lungs loosen up, adrenaline is released. I meditate regularly and see how it makes me feel. But I'm still too much in my head. The body is still underexposed. Through my pregnancy and childbirth, I have become aware that the body is something wonderful, it is brilliantly put together, amazing what I can do with it."

Then we talk about applying for the mandate of the Council of not endorsed spiritual care. "There was a practical reason: otherwise, I would have had to study theology, and I thought I was sufficiently educated. There are things from the church that I can't connect with. For example, there is the status of women in the church, the vision of the ministry, a rigid conception of spirituality that is far away from me. I don't think you have to be religious to live a good life. I also find refusing communion to divorced people an example of putting rules first instead of people."

Anna found the application process at the RING a challenge. "I only had half a year of experience. I spent a lot of time trying to figure out how to word my personal spiritual biography. In the end I found it very vulnerable to write down and at the same time I learned a lot from it. Later I found many more things I could have written. If I had applied a few years later, the process might have gone faster." The assessment, accounting for one's own spirituality for others, was not difficult at all for Anna. She thought it was an opportunity to justify it clearly to herself and not at all too extensive. Her conclusion: "It has been a nice search". The comments she received were to the point. "It said that I had worded my biography well. They could not imagine that I had not yet experienced tension in contact with residents or colleagues. Now I realize that this does not necessarily have to be a conflict, but perhaps just a realization that I am dealing with something completely different."

Is Anna spiritually competent? "I think it's about whether you can recharge your batteries spiritually, find new strength, inspiration and connection. And that you can reflect on that. I think I can do that: I have enough sources of power from which I can drink and from which I can draw energy, sources that are meaningful to me. And I can reflect on that." The professional association has a formal definition of spiritual competence (mentioned in next section). Anna says she could never explain it so specifically, "but from the way I see spirituality I miss in that definition that which makes you warm, where your heart can bloom, where strength emanates from and that this emanates from you, that you make the connection with the higher, with the other, with yourself. It is not a one-way street; it is a connection that you make yourself and how you deal with it." With this statement, Anna agrees with the characterization of spirituality as a living transformation process, a characterization by Waaijman (2000) that has been adopted by the professional association: "The concept of spirituality refers to processes of inner transformation. [. . .] Spirituality concerns our whole being, as it is more about attitude than about a specific domain. It is dynamic rather than static and it touches on questions of meaning and the experience of meaning" (Waajman 2000, 421–22).

For Anna, the personal and the professional are intertwined. "In the work there is a connection from heart-to-heart – or from soul to soul, also a nice word – and that is inextricably linked to me because I am there at that moment who enters into that connection at that moment. And then I draw from my own experience, my life story, from my own sources, to deal with the story that the other person offers me. Even if I follow the other, I always have to be there myself." This is also reflected in the way of praying with people. "I always explain it to people, what do you want us to pray, do you want to pray the Lord's Prayer together, shall I pray for you or do you want to pray alone In this way you arrive at something that you share together, but I always keep my own language, my own feeling." When Anna prays herself – not every day or at every meal – it really is in a different way than she would do with residents.

But there is no break in between. "I always take a piece of Anna with me, even if I do it differently at home. People's expectations don't always match who I'm at home with." Anna could not see herself as a Catholic or Protestant chaplain. She prefers to work in a diverse environment, "where you can develop your own space and move with the rest and the rest with you." She is pleased that a Council for Institutionally Non-Endorsed Spiritual Caregivers has been set up. "It is in line with the trend that people are less and less connected to a church. You respond to a vision of the future in the Netherlands, in fact, in the whole of Western Europe.

As a spiritual caregiver, you are open to all people in the care institution, regardless of their and my background. I would like to see spiritual care less concerned with faith, but more with meaning and spirituality. The church plays no role in the work I do." That is why Anna does not want to advertise herself as a chaplain. "As a believer I know that I can turn to a chaplain, but as a spiritual caregiver, I go beyond faith."

Looking back, it is striking that Anna is exemplary for students of spiritual care today. She has been religiously socialised to a limited extent. The interest in studying religious studies was partly due to how she encountered expressions of worldview in the culture surrounding her. In this way she develops a personal spirituality, which is also characterised as 'worldview bricolage'. Anna considers herself to be just as spiritually competent as her colleagues who receive a mission from the Church. For all kinds of reasons, she does not want to work on behalf of a church and values her autonomy very much. We reflect in more detail on the latter two elements, spiritual competence and autonomy.

5 Spiritual Competence: Representative and Health Professional

Combining the terms "spirituality" and "competence" is disputed by some. After all, competence belongs to the domain of knowledge, skills and attitudes to be developed through education. Spirituality could not be included in that; it is not something that people develop on their own initiative. Spirituality arises in a relationship between human and the divine, in which one opens oneself receptively to the working of grace.[1] Nevertheless, the professional association has chosen in its professional standard to describe 'spiritual competence' as follows: "The ability to help people discover and renew sources of spirituality and belief. This competence is based on a broad knowledge of such sources, and the ability to adapt and present them where necessary in rituals and symbolic ways of expression." Two aspects are central to this description: on the one hand, knowledge of spiritual sources and, on the other hand, the skill to apply this in contact with clients, in conversation and ritual. Spiritual competence is limited to the micro-level in this definition. Earlier, following Cooper-White, we distinguished four levels on

1 For example, in the United Kingdom people prefer to talk about spiritual 'formation', to indicate that this is not about objectively determined learning goals, but that personal integration is desirable.

which spiritual competence can be situated (Smeets and Morice-Calkhoven 2015). Only when a spiritual caregiver 'masters' all these levels can one speak of a spiritual care competency as a whole. The four elements are listed in Table 1.

Table 1: Elements of spiritual (care) competency.

Spiritual competency means:		Level
1	For spiritual caregivers to have a grounded and lived personal worldview identity	Person
2	For spiritual caregivers to be able to relate the patient's story and present situation to his or her worldview identity and spiritual resources	Professional practice
3	For spiritual care to have a professional identity and domain that is clearly defined and distinguished from other professions	Professional identity
4	For spiritual care to be recognised and legitimated at a societal and legal level	Legitimisation

Spiritual competence starts at the level of the person of the spiritual caregiver, to have a grounded and lived personal worldview identity. This identity is not static but dynamic, as we previously referred to spirituality with Waaijman as a permanent inner transformation. At the level of the professional practice, the hermeneutic ability to relate a patient's present experience to his spiritual resources occupies a central position. This is the level that is addressed in the definition of the professional union. Widening the scope to the professional identity as such, the notion of spiritual competence should make clear what uniquely distinguishes spiritual caregivers from other (healthcare) professionals, such as psychotherapists or social workers. And all this ought to result – at the societal and legal level – in the position of spiritual care in society and in the law to be recognized and legitimated. All these four levels together form the competence to practice spiritual care. Our empirical research confirms the four elements of spiritual care competence as a base to guide further reflection and research (Smeets and Morice-Calkhoven 2015). We hope that this broader definition will be included in the proposed revision of the current professional standard of the VGVZ (2015), which was also assessed by Smit (2019) as too individualistic neoliberal.

In the interview, Anna emphasised the first level mentioned above, that of personal spirituality. She misses that in the definition of the professional association. However, the professional association does refer to this level elsewhere. The spiritual caregiver is expected to be "a bearer of one's own religious or worldview sources" (VGVZ 2015, 17). Anna considers this personal aspect to be the basis from which acting in contact with clients (the second level) takes shape. Anna also speaks of the ability to reflect on spirituality. This reflection can relate to all levels: reflection on personal spirituality (level 1), on communication with clients (level 2), on communication and cooperation with other healthcare professionals (level 3), on communication to legitimize one's own domain (level 4). In short, according to Anna, spiritual competence consists of spiritual resourcing and spiritual reflection.

To clarify this further, we can turn to Huijzer (2017). Based on his research among Protestant spiritual caregivers, he arrives at two central concepts: attestation (based on Paul Ricoeur) and integration. On the one hand, the contribution of the spiritual caregiver is a personal testimony, which gives each meeting its own colour. Attestation assumes a 'lived spirituality' through resourcing. A testimony has a linguistically different character than a proclamation. According to De Jong, testimony is the appropriate style to communicate with interlocutors who have a different worldview background (De Jong 2019; Smeets 2020). Attestation, according to Huijzer, should be the character of the communication with clients, based of course on reflection on one's own spirituality. The concept of integration relates to the third and fourth levels of spiritual competence: the interaction with other care providers and the accountability of one's own profession. Here the spiritual caregiver speaks a different language, namely the language of care. This requires meta-reflection on the attestative spiritual communication with clients. And with regard to the inter-worldview aspect, Walton notes that spiritual care should be characterized by a substantive pluriform determination of identity and for respecting the pluriformity of worldview and culture.

The professional attestation as testimony should guarantee dialogue, inclusion and participation (Walton 2020). Or, as Walton says elsewhere: "Diversity is first of all a gift of creation to be celebrated. There is both undeniable communality and irreducible diversity in humanity. Only seeking communalities neutralizes rather than recognizing the differences. Only emphasizing difference makes interreligious and intercultural communication impossible. Absolutizing either commonality or difference can be violent. There is simultaneous sameness and otherness." (Walton 2021, 61). The personal testimony in its aspect of 'sameness' of the spiritual caregiver will therefore always be related to the existing worldview traditions because no one develops their own spirituality in a vacuum. The denominations hope that their tradition is represented in contact with clients. General spiritual caregivers will not want or be able to do this but will always refer to this representation in some way in their testimony, even if only in partial or complete rejection of it. However, their attestation will mainly emphasize the unique otherness in relation to worldview traditions and in this way also support the unique otherness of the clients' personal spirituality and its development during one's biography (Schweitzer 1998). However, in this, they operate no differently than denominational spiritual caregivers, who must also pay attention to clients' own interpretation of spirituality. Viewed in this way, general and denominational spiritual caregivers might be able to come closer together in the future and, in addition to differences, also recognize similarities in everyone's approach.

6 Autonomy in Christian Culture and in Professional Action

Again and again, Anna emphasizes that she makes her own choices with regard to education, with regard to the way in which she does her work and that she shapes her own spirituality. She is the one who chose this education, while her parents were satisfied with an experience of cultural Catholicism. It is she who connects with the client. It is she who makes the connection with herself, the other and the Higher. The autonomous self-awareness that characterizes her and many of her so called 'general' colleagues may raise the question of whether freedom is not over-hyped here. In a workshop of this sector, questions were asked about the desirable designation of this group. The terms independent and unattached came to prominence. The other spiritual caregivers are bound by the vision and regulations of the worldview organization that sends them.

Is this perhaps a false dichotomy? At least for the spiritual caregivers who belong to the Christian and humanistic sector, their culture is also steeped in emancipation and individualization. In his book 'Inventing the individual', Larry Siedentop shows how a movement towards freedom can be recognized in Christian history. He sketches a line that starts with Paul and continues via Augustine to the Middle Ages, to figures such as William of Ockham. "For freedom He has set us free", says Paul, thus supporting the liberation struggle of slaves in Roman culture. With his introspective view, Augustine is one of the founders of thinking about freedom. "For Augustine, the conscious action of the individual has now to be understood as a mysterious merger of intellect and feeling, the result of an obscure process in which the heart is 'stirred'" (Siedentop 2014, 103). In line with this tradition is the Franciscan foreman William of Ockham. For him, it is clear: "God's creation cannot be 'second-guessed'. We have not created ourselves, but we have been created with free will. [. . .] By emphasizing the role of the will, Ockham associated reason with individual experience and choice rather than with 'legislating' about a timeless 'nature' of things [. . .]. Ockham's understanding of justice emerged as the claim for 'equal liberty'. Freedom became a birthright, a right founded on the nature of human agency." (Siedentop 2014, 307, 309, 313). No matter how much the leadership of the Catholic Church, supported by theologians, tries to counter this pursuit of freedom, it is unstoppable. Later, Martin Luther will continue this line in the Reformation by giving the believer the right to his own reading and interpretation of the Bible. In every age, there are Christian inspirations for the pursuit of freedom, with liberation theology as the most recent example.

In the work of spiritual caregivers, one can speak of professional autonomy. In a critical dialogue with the regulatory burden of the bureaucratic care organization on the one hand and with that of the authorities in worldview organizations, the spiritual caregiver takes his own responsibility. The choice not to be sent by a Christian church does not mean that one considers the church irrelevant, but that one does not want to let one's own room for action be determined by an external organization. People do want to account for themselves, but then in dialogue with colleagues, as Anna also witnessed: that is precisely what is emphasized as positive and stimulating for one's own development. But also, for Christian spiritual caregivers, who are sent by the churches, we can say that the development of their freedom does not contradict the Christian tradition.

7 Implications for Education: From CPE (Clinical Pastoral Education) Towards CSE (Clinical Spiritual Education) – A Paradigm Shift Within CPE

Anna followed the CPE in Nijmegen in a spiritually diverse group. "There was never a real clash, I found it very fascinating. I've learned the most from the students closest to me, if only to expose my own allergies and irritations. Things have also become clearer to me that I have always seen very differently." Learning in freedom is one of the characteristics of CPE, not coincidentally also the title of a book by Carl Rogers, one of the founders of humanistic psychology and the inspirer of the 'learning by doing' practice in the CPE courses.

Other students of the training in which Anna participated also had the same experience. Two of them also devote their portfolio reports to it. Gisela writes about how she can reshape her responsibility as a chaplain by illuminating it, inspired by Irvin Yalom (2017), from the existential freedom of human beings: "My personal point of departure in the CPE training was that I sometimes carry too much responsibility. An important learning point is that it also allows me to take responsibility away from others. And that it makes me freer when I can better distinguish between my own responsibility and that of the other. Responsibility and freedom are not always in balance in my ministry and in my private life. You could see my learning goal as a focused search for a better balance between the two. Yalom offers me a new perspective in this. He does not take his starting point in someone's responsibility, but in the freedom of 'authorship'. To be aware of this means to be aware that a person creates his or her own living conditions. That still needs nuance, but the emphasis on the choices that everyone makes in his or her existence shifts my attention from my own sense of responsibility to a constructive interpretation of the word responsibility. Not from a must, but from the existential question of how we as people in this world can learn to use our freedom in such a way that we respond to it in what we do and what we don't do. And how I, as a chaplain, can play a guiding role in this."

The development of the spiritual caregiver's freedom is not the same as the development of a stronger ego. It is about developing an inner freedom, of the person who can look at himself and reality from a distance. Ludwig writes about this in his portfolio: "The 'I' – in the spiritual tradition also called 'self' to distinguish it from 'ego' – which undertakes this passive activity, I would rather not refer to as a 'transcendent I' (in the Eastern, Platonic and Christian sense), but as 'transcendental I' (in a more philosophical sense, though the meaning I give it does not coincide with that of Immanuel Kant). The transcendental self is 'the perceiving mind' within us, an aspect of the human mind that we can better develop through meditation."

Participants also have the same experience in an interprofessional training on meaning in 'listening with space'. One participant testifies that starting from freedom gives her more strength and self-confidence to be close to the other and to use her own talents. These examples illustrate that spiritual competence and freedom are challenges for spiritual caregivers of all denominations. The interreligious dialogue has a broadening and deepening effect. Moreover, spiritual competence and freedom are not only relevant for spiritual caregivers, but for all professionals who want to enter the field of meaning and spirituality and who are seeking training. With this in mind, we are preparing refresher training for interprofessional sense-giving care in Nijmegen. In my opinion, all this implies that the name 'Clinical Pastoral Education' needs to be reconsidered. The main question is whether the word 'Pastoral' still covers the profession sufficiently: the training is not only relevant for Christian chaplains, but for all spiritual caregivers. And it is not only relevant for spiritual counsellors, but for all 'meaning making professionals' (as we see in the European and international context, in the participation of, for example, psychologists, therapists, doctors, psychiatrists, social workers and nurses).

With this in mind, the content of the CPE courses should also be reviewed. Acquiring spiritual competency requires learning activities in each of the four domains listed earlier. The current CPE courses are mainly located at levels 1 and 2. We are thinking of the following elements: a narrative approach in care and counselling (level 2); dealing with meaning and spirituality at the meso-level – because sociocultural processes of secularization, deinstitutionalization and individualization have also become visible in healthcare institutions, affecting both clients, staff and spiritual caregivers. This also concerns the development of administrative and managerial skills, in cooperation with colleagues and within the professional association, and the pursuit of humanization in care and society (levels 3 and 4; cf. Burke 2021, 191–201) and finally, a personal spiritual biography (level 1). The person nowadays is seen as a 'dialogical self' that incorporates different voices. In the biography, participants conduct an internal dialogue, where social and personal elements go together. It forms the basis for the development of contemplative listening to narratives of clients, in which the professional gives a non-evaluative space for dealing with personal and social spiritual dynamics, moral issues and conflicts.

To integrate all these elements in the CPE courses, we need 'models of practice' to develop spiritual competence and spiritual autonomy. There are examples from abroad that we want to be inspired by (e.g., Switzerland, Australia). The implementation of this substantive innovation will probably lead to a paradigm shift: from Clinical Pastoral Education towards Clinical Spiritual Education.

References

Bernts, Ton, and Joantine Berghuijs. 2016. *God in Nederland: 1966–2015*. 1st ed. Utrecht: Ten Have.

Burke, Andree. 2021. 'Sorgen um das Menschliche – Wie Seelsorger*innen sich am gesellschaftlichen Zusammenhalt beteiligen (können)'. *Wege zum Menschen* 73 (3): 191–201. https://doi.org/10.13109/weme.2021.73.3.191.

De Jong, Aad 2019. *Getuigen van de Geest. Een Praktisch-Theologische Benadering van Interreligieuze Dialoog*. Den Haag: Koninklijke Bibliotheek.

Den Draak, Christien, and Wim Smeets, eds. 2010. *Van Kapucijn Tot Consulent Spirituele Zorg. Biografische Ontwikkelingslijnen Bij Veertig Jaar Geestelijke Verzorging*. Tillburg: KSGV.

Huijzer, Richart. 2017. *De Binnenkant van Het Ambt*. Delft: Eburon.

Liefbroer, Anke I, and Joantine Berghuijs. 2017. 'Religieuze En Levensbeschouwelijke Diversiteit in Het Werk van Geestelijk Verzorgers'. *Tijdschrift Geestelijke Verzorging* 20 (3): 24–33.

Napel-Roos, Nelleke ten, Brenda Mathijssen, Wim Smeets, and Hetty Zock. 2021. 'Non-Denominational Spiritual Care Givers and the Development of Their Spirituality.' *Health & Social Care Chaplaincy* 9 (1): 60–79. https://doi.org/10.1558/hscc.40706.

Puchalski, Christina M, Betty Ferrell, Rose Virani, Shirley Otis-Green, Pamela Baird, Janet Bull, Harvey Chochinov, et al. 2009. 'Improving the Quality of Spiritual Care as a Dimension of Palliative Care: The Report of the Consensus Conference'. *Journal of Palliative Medicine* 12 (10): 885–904. https://doi.org/10.1089/jpm.2009.0142.

Schweitzer, Friedrich. 1998. *Die Suche nach eigenem Glauben. Einführung in die Religionspädagogik des Jugendalters.* Gütersloh: Chr. Kaiser Gütersloher Verlagshaus.
Siedentop, Larry. 2014. *Inventing the Individual: The Origins of Western Liberalism*. 1st ed. Cambridge (Mass.): Harvard University Press.
Smeets, Wim. 2020. 'Zinervaring in gesprek'. *Religie & Samenleving* 15 (3): 257–86. https://doi.org/10.54195/RS.11501.
Smeets, Wim, F W J Gribnau, and Johannes van der Ven. 2011. 'Quality Assurance and Spiritual Care'. *Journal of Empirical Theology* 24 (1): 80–121.
Smeets, Wim, and Tessa Morice-Calkhoven. 2015. 'From Ministry Towards Spiritual Competence. Changing Perspectives in Spiritual Care in the Netherlands'. In *The Concept of Religion. Defining and Measuring Contemporary Beliefs and Practices*, edited by H Schilderman, 103–29. Leiden: Brill.
Smit, Job. 2019. 'Met Geestelijke Verzorging Verder. Een Kritische Blik Op de Beroepsstandaard'. *Tijdschrift Geestelijke Verzorging* 22 (95): 24–31.
VGVZ. 2015. *Beroepsstandaard*. Utrecht: VGVZ.
Waajman, Kees. 2000. *Spiritualiteit. Vormen, Grondslagen, Methoden*. Utrecht: Kok.
Walton, Martin. 2020. 'Meerduidig en meervoudig: Interreligieuze en interculturele dialoog in geestelijke verzorging'. *Religie & Samenleving* 15 (3): 240–56. https://doi.org/10.54195/RS.11500.
Walton, Martin. 2021. 'Encountering Difference. Repertoire of Intercultural and Interreligious Chaplaincy'. In *Care, Healing and Human Well-Being within Interreligious Discourses*, edited by Helmut Weiss, Karl H Federschmidt, Daniël Louw, and Lidna Sauer Bredvik, 51–65. Stellenbosch: African Sun Media.
Yalom, Irvin D. 2017. *Becoming Myself: A Psychiatrist's Memoir*. London: Little Brown Book.
Zock, Hetty. 2019. 'Chaplaincy in the Netherlands: The Search for a Professional and a Religious Identity'. *Tidsskrift for Praktisk Teologi* 36 (2): 11–21. https://doi.org/10.48626/tpt.v36i2.5347.

Author Biographies

Michael Balboni is an Instructor at Harvard Medical School and a congregational minister at a downtown church in Boston, Massachusetts. As a social scientist, his empirical projects focus on spirituality and religion in serious illness, including among patients, clinicians, and religious communities. He is published two books, including *Hostility to Hospitality* (Oxford 2019), and *Spirituality and Religion within the Culture of Medicine* (Oxford 2017). He serves as a pastor to healthcare professionals within an intentional Christian community, and cares for many congregants within a large urban congregation.

Tracy Balboni holds degrees from Stanford University, Harvard Medical School and the Harvard School of Public Health and is board certified in both radiation oncology and palliative medicine. Dr. Balboni currently serves as Professor of Radiation Oncology at Harvard Medical School and as Program Director of the Harvard Radiation Oncology Program. She also co-leads the Initiative on Health, Religion, and Spirituality at Harvard University. Dr. Balboni's primary research interests are located at the intersection of oncology, palliative care, and the role of spirituality in life-threatening illness. This includes the impact of religion/spirituality on coping and end-of-life medical care and the impact of spiritual care in the medical setting on patient end-of-life outcomes.

Annette Haußmann is Professor of Practical Theology with focus on Pastoral and Spiritual Care at Heidelberg University. She is Scientific Director of the Center for Pastoral Care of the Protestant regional Church in Baden that offers pastoral care education and further trainings. As a licensed psychological psychotherapist (CBT) her research interests involve the relation of psychotherapy, pastoral/spiritual care, the entanglement of mental health and religion/sprituality. The primarily empirical research also addresses the role of caring communities in health and social care, family caregiving and religion/spirituality, and volunteering in pastoral caregiving.

Trace Haythorn is the former executive director of ACPE, the Association for Clinical Pastoral Education. Today he serves as an executive coach and consultant, bringing 25 years of leadership to service with people and organizations across the US. Out of his love for spiritual care and his deep belief in its potential to heal the world, Trace continues to work with the Chaplaincy Innovation Lab, Transforming Chaplaincy, the George Washington Institute for Spirituality and Health (GWish), City of Hope's ICC program, and the European Research Institute for Chaplains in Healthcare (ERICH).

David Neuhold is Professor for Church History at the University of Lucerne. He studied Physics and Catholic Theology in Graz (Austria) and Fribourg and holds a Doctorate (Second Vatican Council) and a Habilitation (Sacred Heart Devotion) in Church History. He was a Research Associate at the SZRKG/RSHRC (Swiss Journal of Religious and Cultural History) and at the Professorship for Spiritual Care at the University of Zurich, where he published (together with Simon Peng-Keller) the volume "*Charting Spiritual Care. The Emerging Role of Chaplaincy Records in Global Health Care*" (2020).

Daniel Nuzum is an adjunct lecturer at the College of Medicine and Health at University College Cork (UCC) alongside his work as a healthcare chaplain, Clinical Pastoral Education supervisor and educator with a specialist interest in perinatal care, pregnancy loss, palliative care and bereavement care. Dr. Nuzum received his PhD from University College Cork in 2016 with a thesis entitled '*The spiritual and professional impact of stillbirth*'. Daniel is an active member of the Pregnancy Loss

https://doi.org/10.1515/9783112205839-012

Research Group at UCC. Daniel has published and presented in the areas of perinatal bereavement, communication, stillbirth, palliative care and spiritual care. Daniel's research interests are in the area of care following stillbirth and neonatal bereavement, spirituality in specialist palliative care, pastoral education and healthcare ethics. Daniel lectures on the undergraduate medical programme on whole person care and communication skills and on the MSc in Palliative care at UCC.

Simon Peng-Keller is Professor for Spiritual Care at the Faculty of Theology and the Study of Religion at the University of Zurich. Alongside his academic work, he is also engaged in contemplative retreats and was healthcare chaplain at the centre for palliative care at the University Hospital of Zurich. His main areas of research are interprofessional spiritual care, palliative care, visionary experience near death, theology of spirituality and Christian contemplation.

Traugott Roser, a Protestant pastor, has been a Professor of practical theology with a focus on pastoral care, spiritual and palliative care as well as liturgy and pastoral theology at the University of Münster since 2013. Between 2010 and 2013, he held Europe's first endowed professorship for spiritual care at the medical faculty of the LMU Munich. Previously, he worked as a pastor in the fields of palliative care, hospitals and retirement homes. He is an appointed member of the Bavarian Ethics Council, the Ethics Committee of the Medical Association of Westphalia-Lippe, the Standing Conference for Pastoral Care at the Council of the EKD, the Liturgical Conference of the EKD and the Theological Committee of the Evangelical Church of the Union. In 2021, he was awarded the special prize of the Wichern Prize of Diakonie Germany.

Wim Smeets is a spiritual caregiver in an elderly home and home care in the Netherlands. He is also a CPE-supervisor, associate Professor of 'innovation in spiritual care' at the Radboud University Nijmegen Medical Center and president of the European Council for Pastoral Care and Counseling (ECPCC).

Chris Swift has worked in chaplaincy for 30 years. This has included part-time prison ministry; teaching Masters courses for military chaplains; and a significant period spent in the health and social care sector. His PhD was an exploration of spiritual care in the UK's National Health Service (NHS) and forms the foundation of his title *Hospital Chaplaincy in the Twenty-first Century*. Chris holds an honorary research post at the University of Leeds and was Visiting Professor of Religious, Spiritual and Pastoral Care at Staffordshire University. In 2024 Chris became Director of the Leeds Church Institute, UK.

John Swinton is Professor in Practical Theology and Pastoral Care and Chair in Divinity and Religious Studies at the University of Aberdeen. For more than a decade John worked as a registered mental health nurse. He also worked for a number of years as a hospital and community mental health chaplain alongside people with severe mental health challenges. In 2004, he founded the University of Aberdeen's Centre for Spirituality, Health and Disability. He has published widely within the area of mental health, dementia, disability theology, spirituality and healthcare, end of life care, qualitative research and pastoral care. John is the author of a number of monographs, including his recent book: *Finding Jesus in the Storm: The Spiritual Lives of Christians with Mental Health Challenges* (Eerdmans 2020). His book *Dementia: Living in the Memories of God* won the Archbishop of Canterbury's Ramsey Prize for excellence in theological writing.

Anna Vandenhoeck is associate professor in pastoral care and diakonia and chair of the Academic Centre for Practical Theology at the Faculty of Theology and Religious Studies, KU Leuven. Her research focuses on pastoral care and spiritual care in health care. She has contributed to spiritual care studies and chaplaincy studies through several books and articles. She is director of the European Research Institute for Chaplains in Healthcare (ERICH) and has been the coordinator of the European Network for Healthcare Chaplains (ENHCC). Anne teaches generalist spiritual care to students in psychology, medicines, physiotherapy, and specialist spiritual care to students in theology. She is part of the international faculty of ISPEC at George Washington Institute for Spirituality and Health, USA.

Fabian Winiger studied medical anthropology at the University of Oxford and at the University of Hong Kong. He is a Senior Research Fellow at the Professorship for Spiritual Care at the University of Zurich, where he conducts research on health and spirituality in the WHO and other United Nations agencies. As part of the URPP Digital Religion(s), Dr. Fabian Winiger investigates spiritual care in digital healthcare settings.